Communicating Trauma

M000202873

Communicating Trauma explores the various aspects of language and communication and how their development can be affected by childhood trauma and overwhelm. Multiple case-study vignettes describe how different kinds of childhood trauma can manifest in children's ability to relate, attend, learn, and communicate. These examples offer ways to understand, respond, and support children who are communicating overwhelm. In this book, psychotherapists, speech-language pathologists, social workers, educators, occupational and physical therapists, medical personnel, foster parents, adoption agencies, and other child professionals and caregivers will find information and practical direction for improving connection and behavior, reducing miscommunication, and giving a voice to those who are often our most challenging children.

Na'ama Yehuda, MSC, SLP, is a speech-language pathologist and audiologist with over 25 years' experience. A clinician in private practice, she consulted for the New York City Department of Education; provides international professional development and consultations on communication, language, trauma, and development; and is the author of several publications on the topic. She was elected to serve on the boards of directors of the Israeli Speech Hearing Language Association (ISHLA) and the International Society for the Study of Trauma and Dissociation (ISSTD), chairs and volunteers on task forces and committees, and co-chairs the Child and Adolescent Committee of ISSTD. She also writes and publishes fiction.

Communicating Trauma

Clinical Presentations and Interventions
with Traumatized Children

Na'ama Yehuda

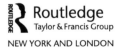
Routledge
Taylor & Francis Group

NEW YORK AND LONDON

First published 2016
by Routledge
711 Third Avenue, New York, NY 10017

and by Routledge
2 Park Square, Milton Park, Abingdon, Oxon OX14 4RN

Routledge is an imprint of the Taylor & Francis Group, an informa business

Library of Congress Cataloging-in-Publication Data
Yehuda, Na'ama.
   Communicating trauma : clinical presentations and interventions with traumatized children / Na'ama Yehuda. — 1 Edition.
      pages cm
   Includes bibliographical references and index.
   1. Psychic trauma in children—Treatment.   2. Child development.   3. Communication.   I. Title.
   RJ506.P66Y44 2016
   618.92'8521—dc23
   2015013577

ISBN: 978-0-415-74309-9 (hbk)
ISBN: 978-0-415-74310-5 (pbk)
ISBN: 978-1-315-81386-8 (ebk)

Typeset in Minion
by Apex CoVantage, LLC

For a little girl
With yellow hair
And for children
Everywhere

Contents

Acknowledgments

This book would never have been written if it were not for my clients. My first thanks go to the children and their families in all their configurations and presentations. They are steadfast teachers and continue to educate me, each in his or her unique way of communicating and relating. This book is really theirs: a product of the questions they raised in me and which sent me searching for what else might be going on and the skills I needed to help them better; of the feelings they communicated and evoked in me; of the actions that spoke volumes even when there were no words. To all my clients, past and present, you have my gratitude.

Thanks go to my friends and colleagues at my professional homes at ISHLA (Israeli Speech Hearing Language Association), and ISSTD (the International Society for the Study of Trauma and Dissociation), my colleagues on the Child and Adolescent Committee, and my friends at ISSTDNYC—too numerous to list, yet the source of many friendships. Special thanks to Dr. Joy Silberg for opening the door at ISSTD and to Fran Waters and Sandra Baita for warm friendships and expertise. To my sister Dr. Ruth Rosen-Zvi, clinical child psychologist: for consults, venting, and more. To my friend and colleague of thirty years Ronit Koren and to Dr. Tova Most and Dr. Etti Dromi of Tel-Aviv University, professors extraordinaire and supporters of all my professional adventures. To my TT friends: for the profound healing of centering and compassion.

Thank you to Anna Moore, senior editor at Routledge, for the seed of this book and for being there for every query, and to the rest of the staff at Routledge, turning draft manuscripts into books: I love this magic.

Very special thanks go to Dr. Adele Ryan McDowell, an always-there cheerleader, good juju sender, and mentor; to Jenny Heinz, a better attuned clinician no one can find: Your love amazes me. To my incredible friends and loved ones, so understanding of my 'hibernation' when I was busy writing: my brilliant family; my mom Riva Yehuda and my sisters Tamar, Michal, Hadasa, Yael, Shulamit, and Ruth; my nieces and nephews, grand-nieces and grand-nephews—you are tremendous blessings. Last but not least, soul-kisses to Carol Hornig and Kathryn Cameron—I know the two of you watch over me and over the children who did not make it. I love you more.

Preface

Timothy was two. He used few intelligible sounds, was fussy, and had feeding issues and high sensitivity in his mouth. He got overwhelmed easily and would stop responding, shake, and lose muscle tone. Born prematurely, Timothy underwent many medical procedures during the first few weeks of his life.

Martina spoke with a noticeable lisp and high-pitched, breathy voice. The nine-year-old had language-learning delays, along with attention and memory difficulties, 'daydreaming,' and irritability. She had severe asthma and lived in a poorly maintained housing project where she was constantly exposed to roaches and rodents.

Leila, age six, had language-learning delay and attention issues. She also had mercurial mood shifts, memory issues, and difficulties understanding how actions and consequences connected. She was diagnosed with ADHD and "probably bipolar," and was described as a "good-child/devil-child." She lived in multiple foster-homes after being removed from her mother's care due to severe childhood neglect and abuse.

Shlomy, age three and a half, spoke in short utterances and was behind expectations in many measures of communication. He "did not listen well," threw tantrums when misunderstood, and was 'expelled' from nursery school for biting. His mother had debilitating postpartum depression after his birth and struggled to care for him through the first six months of his life.

Early trauma—especially chronic and multifaceted—affects children's development. Children can be traumatized by maltreatment (abuse and/or neglect), as well as by invasive and painful medical interventions and chronic illness, by witnessing domestic violence and parental overwhelm, by accidents and disasters, by grief, loss, war, and terror. Communication disorders, disabilities, and delays place children at a high risk for maltreatment and attachment issues, as well as increase the likelihood of frustration and distress. In some children, such as those born prematurely, after intrauterine exposures, or with sensory integration and processing issues, regulatory systems can be less effective and more easily overwhelmed, further complicating reactions to stress.

Even adults with well-formed language abilities often struggle to verbalize distress, let alone children—whose communicative abilities are still forming.

Rather than verbally, many children communicate their distress in how they behave, how they relate to others, how they react, respond, remember, and learn. Traumatized children often present with delays and difficulties in attending and learning, as well as with behavioral and social issues. They are more likely to require special education and are at a higher risk of repeating grades, dropping out of school, getting in trouble, and being diagnosed with mental illness. Trauma can have profound impact on children's presentation and communicative functioning, yet there's relatively little clinical information on the particular ways in which duress manifests in children's language and communication; or on how to best support these in them. When trauma is not directly assessed, children can accumulate hosts of diagnoses that try to account for their myriad symptoms: ADHD, bipolar disorder, autism, auditory processing disorder, conduct disorder, childhood psychosis, and more.

Speech-language pathologists and audiologists are at the forefront of identifying, diagnosing, and treating communication disorders and delays. These include issues with language content and usage; hearing, listening, attending, discriminating, identifying, processing, learning, comprehending, and expressing; as well as articulation, voice, and speech. They may be the first professionals to see children whose learning or communication skills lag behind those of their peers. Because many children experience trauma, and given how disabilities increase risks further, the clinical presentation of many referred children may be affected by trauma. However, communication-disorder clinicians and other child professionals often do not have the training to recognize, account for, or address the impact of trauma and dissociation.

Similarly, many mental health professionals are not aware of the ways trauma impacts children's communication and/or development; even though language and communication are part of many therapeutic interventions, narrative, and interpretation of feelings and events. Lack of information can result in misunderstanding children's abilities and difficulties. It can fragment and misdirect treatment and may limit professionals' ability to respond effectively to a child's needs. Pediatric clinicians, caregivers, and educators all play a role in identification, referral, and treatment of traumatized children, and can benefit from informed collaboration. This manuscript hopes to help with that.

Communicating Trauma explores the co-occurrence, possible relationship, and presentation of communication disorders and posttraumatic/dissociative disorders in traumatized children. It touches on various aspects of neurodevelopment and the ways they are impacted by trauma, stress, and overwhelm, along with the role of attachment and life experiences in language and communication development. The relevance of trauma understanding for speech-language pathologists, education professionals, medical personnel, physical and occupational therapists, social workers, foster-parents, adoption agencies, and other child professionals is discussed, as are the benefits of collaboration. The children themselves taught me most, and so interwoven into the text are numerous vignettes from case-studies culled from over 25 years of clinical work in communication disorders in pediatric populations. Some details and identifying information were changed to maintain client confidentiality, but these cases represent real clinical presentations following various trauma histories. I included narratives from therapeutic interactions with children, educators, clinicians, and caregivers to illustrate examples of psychoeducation, practical solutions, and dilemmas. Suggestions for assessment and intervention for everyday and therapeutic interactions are listed, too.

Part 1 provides a brief overview of communication, language, attachment, and relating, along with the main 'stages' of language acquisition and its social use. Part 2 details the various paths to trauma and traumatic impact in children—from the indirect trauma of prematurity, chronic pain, and caregiver overwhelm to the direct harm of neglect and abuse and the deleterious effects of chronic stress on growth and regulation. In Part 3, the ways trauma can impact language, attention and learning, vocabulary and semantics, pragmatics and socialization are detailed, along with their clinical implications. Part 4 follows with the clinical presentation of communication disorders in traumatized children and the various aspects of assessment that may be relevant to bear in mind. Part 5 deals with intervention recommendations and practical considerations. Marcus (Chapters 8 and 16) once told me: "Sometimes books help." For him and others, I hope this one does.

Part 1

A Brief Overview of Communication, Language, and Development

1 Infant Communication and Attachment

Reciprocity, Verbalization, and Regulation

Billy, age nine months, shrieks when he sees his dad. He lifts his arms and babbles: "Da-da-da!" His father smiles widely, puts down his briefcase, and approaches the baby. "Hi'ya, Billy boy! Nice to see you, too! Want a spin?" He lifts the infant in the air and twirls around. Billy laughs in delight.

Ricky, age nine months, shrieks when he sees his mother. He lifts his arms and babbles: "Ma-ma-ma!" His mother puts down her bag without letting go of the phone, ". . . so then he says to me . . ." she speaks into it, glancing at Ricky and walking past the infant to the other room. Ricky's face changes from elation to disappointment. He reaches toward his mother's back and cries.

Communication

Communication defines our experience. It is how we interpret and express our reality; how we relate and describe who we are; how we comprehend and perceive others; how we let others know our needs, ideas, and dreams. Communication is so intrinsic to human beings that we do it constantly: in words, in body language, actions, and reactions, even lack of response. We communicate verbally and nonverbally to convey information (e.g. share feelings, explain concepts, answer questions), to express needs and ideas (e.g. request, question, voice thoughts, and plans), and to understand others' communication and needs (Berman 2004, Gleason & Ratner 2009).

Verbal communication includes the words we use, how we put them together into sentences, and our intonation, voice, and intention (e.g. request, question, note, humor, irony). Nonverbal communication encompasses posture and facial expression, gestures, and physical reaction or inaction (e.g. handing a requested item, tears, ignoring). Whether with or without words, nonverbal communication is integral to every face-to-face interaction, conveying information about intensity, mood, agreement, or denial.

In the vignette above, little Billy communicated his delight at the sight of his father in voice and gestures. His father responded in kind, interpreting the infant's motion as a request for connection and interaction. Both infant and adult accentuated their exchange with smiles and happy intonation. Billy was understood. His father felt welcomed. Both experienced pleasant feelings, successful communication, and a reinforcement of their bond.

Little Ricky also communicated his delight at seeing his mother, but his mother's response did not acknowledge the baby's gesture and vocalization. When she walked past him, Ricky's communicative intent failed and his emotions changed from elation to confusion, frustration, and anger. Too young to convey feelings in words, Ricky reacted by crying, which often serves to express amplified need for connection and reassurance (Ninio & Snow 1996).

Communication Failure

Not all interactions are successful or satisfying. Factors such as age and ability affect the end result. Adults often take on the responsibility to decipher a baby's intent, but expect increased clarity and shared responsibility for successful communication as children grow. Errors or ambiguity may be acceptable from a toddler or an ill person, but less so from an older child or a healthy adult. Proficiency, knowledge of social customs, and understanding of symbolic language (idioms, puns, expressions) play a role in how successful communication becomes, as does familiarity with the speaker/s (e.g. a stranger vs. a sibling or friend). Context and place combine with the personalities and abilities of those involved to determine how well intention is conveyed and received, and whether communication succeeded or failed. Access to language and familiarity with its rules scaffold successful communication, which fosters satisfaction, closeness, and ease. Failure, on the other hand, is more likely to lead to embarrassment, awkwardness, confusion, distance, and anger (Gleason & Ratner 2009, Ninio & Snow 1996, Schiefelbusch 1986).

Children's linguistic and cognitive abilities are still developing, which makes them vulnerable to communication failure. In response, adults usually try to infer the child's intent and use modeling and narrative to minimize misunderstandings (Gleason & Ratner 2009, Ninio & Snow 1996). While some frustration is inevitable, an adult's familiarity with the child's routines, preferences, needs, vocalizations, behaviors, and dislikes helps lessen it. However, communication failure is very high for children with developmental and communication difficulties, as it is for young children around adults who do not know them well and for those compromised by illness or pain (Kuttner 2010, Schiefelbusch 1986). For these children, failure might happen often and is compounded by the very issues that had caused it: a small vocabulary, illness and limited attention, comprehension and processing issues, difficulty organizing ideas, unintelligible speech, and insufficient language.

Language

The Merriam-Webster dictionary defines language as "the system of words or signs that people use to express thoughts and feelings to each other . . . the words, their pronunciation, and the methods of combining them used and understood by a community." By definition, language must be shared by at least two people to be utilized for communication (why children deprived of language exposure do not learn to speak). While all languages in the world follow rules of content (vocabulary), form (morphology and syntax), and use (pragmatics), people speaking different languages cannot understand each other. This is because languages have different sound systems and different rules for joining sounds together into words and for stringing words in sentences. The same thing can be referred to by different sound combinations (e.g. /chair/ or /kiseh/ for what one sits on), and identical sound combinations can carry different meanings (e.g. /me/ means "myself" in English but "who" in Hebrew). Languages also differ in how word order appears in sentences, coding for person, tense, gender, number, and possession, familiar versus formal language, etc. Each language includes expressions, metaphors, and social rules for use and meaning. For languages that include written codes, variability extends to sound symbols (e.g. letters or word glyphs), directionality (e.g. left to right), and punctuation (Adams 1994, Gleason & Ratner 2009).

Language Learning

Many people associate language learning with the acquisition of a second (or additional) language, where learners use their knowledge of how language works as scaffolding: They know there will be words to name things, people, actions, and descriptions; they know words will form sentences to express meanings (Bialystok 2001, Erdos et al 2010, Harding & Riley 1986, Talamas et al 1999). The more frequent and universal language learning, however, takes place in infants, who have no model to compare to and are tasked with acquiring language while their cognitive, relational, and developmental abilities are still maturing. Infants must map out the sound system of their language by differentiating which sound variations carry meaning and which do not, what acoustic variation may be semantic (e.g. 'bat'/'bag') or indicate intent (e.g. question/statement) and what represents inter- and intra-speaker variability (loud/soft voice, mom vs. dad). At the same time, infants need to extract meaning from words as well as infer how that meaning changes in context. They should understand that whether visible ("Daddy is home") or invisible ("Daddy went to work"), the meaning of some words (i.e. Daddy) remain the same, while the meaning of other words changes ("He" can be Daddy, or the puppy, or the mailman; "big" can mean the ball, but also the fridge, bus, elephant, and the neighbors' Labrador) (Dromi 1987, Gleason & Ratner 2009). Infants do all that with a cognitive system that is still figuring out the world and everything in it, a motor system that is not yet under their control, and a regulatory system that is still evolving (more on early language development in Chapter 2).

As long as they have sufficient exposure, repetition, and opportunity, along with adequate perception, cognition, and attention, most children manage to acquire language. Exposure is paramount. Children who are not spoken to are left bereft of language. Children's communication is fundamentally impacted and shaped by the exposure experiences they get. The ways others interact with the child and interpret possible perceptions, actions, and feelings in the child affect communication, relating, and how meaning is formed.

Interactive experiences start early. Fetuses can hear during the last trimester of pregnancy. They may respond to voices and tones, and some show recognition of familiar ones after birth (Nazzi et al 1998). Newborns can focus on a caregiver's face immediately after birth. They show sensitivity to mood and intonation and can reflexively reciprocate some facial movements. This mimicking may have relational significance and often reinforces bonding. Newborns' reciprocation is possibly partially neurologically encoded and some researchers attribute it to mirror-neurons (Fogassi & Ferrarri 2007).

Mirror-Neurons and Their Importance to Development

Mirror-neurons were discovered during the study of single neuron activity in the ventral prefrontal cortex of macaque monkeys. Rizzolatti was studying how neurons responded to actions and they found that neurons that 'code' for goal-directed motor movements activated not only when a monkey was doing a grasping action but also when that monkey *observed* a researcher doing a grasping action. Interestingly the neurons activated only if the action was goal directed: Observing a random hand movement did not elicit the neurons' activation, while a similar movement directed at waving 'hello,' did. The correspondence between observed action and premotor neuron activation led to the neurons being labeled "mirror-neurons" (Gaensbauer 2011, Rizzolatti & Craighero 2004).

The discovery of mirror-neurons added to the understanding of children's and adults' capacities to 'embody' observed experience, especially as further research showed that neurons associated with a goal-directed action could be activated by stimuli across multiple sensory modalities. Mirror-neurons' function was demonstrated for imitation, facial emotion processing, social cognition, and empathy. Not only did the neurons activate when the action was done and when the action was observed, but also when other sensory information relating to that action was perceived (Fogassi & Ferrarri 2007, Gaensbauer 2011).

Infants and young children experience the world, their bodies, and the actions of others through their senses. Input from the environment forms the basis for the child's reactions to stimuli later on (Rizzolatti and Craighero 2004, van der Kolk 2014). This makes caregivers' actions and reactions fundamental to children's actions and reactions to the world around them: It is through adults' responses to the infant and the reactions these elicit in the baby that meaning is established. While mirror-neurons do not have a 1:1 connection to the development of response and reaction, they contribute to our understanding of how patterns learned in early childhood become hard-wired. Early patterns of activation reinforce both positive and negative learning experiences. They may explain why a baby for whom hands brought comfort stops crying and responds with reaching toward the person who reaches for her. They may also explain why a child for whom hands meant pain can respond with lashing out even when someone may be reaching to her in kindness. They may explain why a well-cared-for baby smiles back at someone's grin while a maltreated child might look away in wariness (Gaensbauer 2011).

Such learned patterns of response help explain why removing a child from an abusive environment may not be sufficient for changing the child's actions and reactions to the world around him/her. For new patterns to form, patterns formed in earlier interactions need to be addressed, and reparative interactions should be repeatedly introduced so that repetition can reinforce new response. Children who experience repeated calming are generally more adept at calming, while children who experience repeated stress become quite 'adept' at activating stress responses.

Neuronal activation takes place not only when observing an action or carrying out an action, but even when one is simulating the action in his/her mind (Decety et al 2002). An internalized concept becomes part of our response: For those who found hugs comforting, visualizing a hug can help regulate distress, while visualizing being hurt can elicit distress. Such simulation need not be conscious (i.e. aware)—early patterns of response can be activated by reminders of internal representations across sensory modalities (Decety & Chaminade 2003, Gaensbauer 2011). This augments the understanding of how posttraumatic responses can take place long after the environment itself changed. Moreover, neurological connections that were formed during overwhelm can become reinforced every time a trauma reminder activates them, forming increasingly 'efficient' pathways for posttraumatic response.

Neurocognitive Development—Efficiency and Specialization

Brains grow through experience. Babies are born with immature nervous systems that are immensely vulnerable and amazingly flexible. Throughout the first few years of life, neurons get sheathed in myelin to improve processing speed and localization, and novel and reinforced connections weave together areas of the brain. This development allows for efficiency, specialization, modulation, and pruning as areas of the brain take on specialized functions (e.g. finger movement coordination, pitch processing) and as the baby's ability to modulate the intensity of a reaction improves. Underutilized neuronal fibers get pruned while those that get utilized frequently form strong connections (Schore 2012, van der Kolk 2014).

A peek into the internal workings of what happens when little Billy hears his name called by his dad and responds by smiling offers an example for this specialized and reinforced neural network. Activated by the sound, the baby's auditory nerves send the acoustic information weaving through the brainstem and into the auditory cortex. The sound is discriminated from other sounds in the background, and previously formed connections activate the area of his brain involved with memory, identifying the voice as belonging to this caregiver and associating it with sensory and emotive memories of how his dad makes Billy feel. Billy's visual cortex is activated too, activating feedback loops of associations with the dad's face and the integrated memories of the dad's voice. Language areas activate in response to the familiar sound combination (Billy's name) and the tone and intonation it was said in. The recognition further activates the limbic system, and the positive affective association to this sound combination releases neurotransmitters of pleasure, bonding, and well-being. The affective response combined with pathways for smiling interacts with motor areas in both hemispheres. The latter coordinate Billy's facial muscles to generate a smile. The activation of facial muscles in that pattern along with the sensory feedback and its associations flood Billy with more pleasant sensations and anticipation of positive interaction and satisfying care.

This simplified schema of stimuli-and-response is a poor representation for the actual intricacy of interwoven and multiply connected links; all of which become increasingly reinforced as interactions repeat in daily variations and contexts to form complex neural tapestries of perception, reaction, and response. Unfortunately, neural tapestries just as complex can form for less favorable response patterns, too—in babies who associate their caregivers' voice with fear or a smirk with possible pain. Repeated activation of those patterns can become powerfully reinforced by autonomic nervous system reactions for fight or flight, overwhelm and dissociation (Cozolino 2014, Gaensbauer 2011, Siegel 2012, van der Kolk 2014).

Though different areas of the brain develop at different rates depending on age, developmental stage, task, stimulation, genetics, and temperament, the whole brain is involved—and develops—throughout childhood. Connections form among feelings, words, tone, sensations, movement, and more, with both hemispheres undergoing massive specialization and specification. As information crisscrosses back and forth between the hemispheres, the corpus callosum thickens. Intricate connections weave semantics and pitch, intonation and meaning, faces and voices, feelings and sensations, motor coordination and bilateral sensory information. Localization and integration take place as the whole brain becomes literally built by experience, both good and bad (Cozolino 2014, Fogassi & Ferrarri 2007, Gaensbauer 2011, Schore 2012, Siegel 2012, van der Kolk 2014).

The Building Blocks of Communication: Reciprocity, Verbalization, and Regulation

Shira is two minutes old. Wrinkled and red, the wailing newborn was checked, wrapped, and placed in her mother's arms. The two lock eyes. Shira stops wailing, calmed by the swaddling and the familiar beat of her mother's heart. Shira's mother cradles her and gazes at the newborn. Shira gazes back. "There you go . . . all safe and snug. . . aren't you a beauty?" the mother croons, oblivious to medical ministrations still being performed. "Yes, you . . . you!" Shira holds her mother's gaze and her tiny lips purse a circle, mirroring her mother's mouth.

Complex communication already takes place even immediately after birth. Mothers gaze at babies; babies gaze at mothers. We smile and coo, narrate, hum, caress, comment, and sing in undertone. In days following, we narrate what we do as we change newborns' diapers and bathe, dress, and prepare to feed or burp them. We interpret cries, smiles, gurgles, and facial expressions; we put words to what we believe the baby is 'telling us.' On their end, newborns focus on our faces and may calm at our voice. They may mimic facial expressions—perhaps not consciously and yet deeply meaningfully to the parent.

Mere weeks later, babies smile intentionally at the sight and voice of loved ones; make noises; and move arms, legs, and head. They interact. Babies continue to reciprocate interaction throughout their waking hours as they grow: They play peek-a-boo and tug on sleeves, they screech, vocalize, smile, frown, make spit bubbles, and belly laugh. They wait for you to do the funny thing again. They take turns. They reach for and hand over items.

Babies are magnificently adept at interaction, but that development depends on reciprocity. If not talked to, if caregivers do not make repeated eye contact, fail to speak to the baby, or to offer connection—babies will not interact well. In extreme cases (e.g. institutions or severe neglect) babies might not interact at all. Even if the physical needs of the children are provided for, without interaction and opportunities for reciprocity babies might not make eye contact or only do so sporadically. They might not cry or be inconsolable, seem more interested in things than people. They rock. Their communication delayed, they won't know how to interact, how to listen, or how to take turns (Bowlby 1997, Fox et al 1988, Hough & Kaczmarek 2011, Miller 2005).

Interaction and reciprocity develop regulation as well as connection. Routine activities such as diapering, feeding, washing, dressing, taking a walk, or rocking to sleep provide repeated opportunities for regulation. In well-cared-for babies, discomfort is noted, interpreted, accepted, and attended to. The baby learns that discomfort passes and that interaction precedes it. They begin to anticipate care even before the discomfort is gone: A hungry baby may quiet as the mother enters the nursery. Still hungry and uncomfortable, the baby had learned that the mother's arrival signals comfort, and so the baby's stress already begins to regulate. It is the consistent and sensitive assistance of caregivers that enables babies to learn how to regulate their own arousal.

This early self-regulation is further reinforced when the mother smiles at the baby who stopped crying as she entered. The mother's own arousal at the baby's distress is calmed and her comfort and confidence in caring for her baby increases. The baby is praised for patience and the mother communicates acceptance and competence, which further strengthen their bonding and the baby's trust in the mother's calming ministrations. Such minutiae of daily care help lay down pathways for regulation and modulation of affect and arousal— neurologically, emotionally, psychologically, physiologically, and socially.

Autism: A Window to Lack of Reciprocity

Communication requires reciprocity. Lack of sensitive interaction by adults thwarts infant communication, but children are integral to the dyad too. Families of autistic children offer a window into what happens when reciprocity is stunted (Hastings et al 2005, Siller & Sigman 2002, Sussman 1999). Parents might find it difficult to calm a baby who is overly sensitive to sensory stimulation and not comforted by voice or touch, who does not respond, or who screams louder when rocked and held. Feeling ill equipped and with their communications unrewarded, parents' own arousal—stress, worry, fatigue, guilt, frustration— may be harder to regulate as interactions become stressful. Even when calm, the baby may not return eye contact and 'look right through' the parent. Objects may elicit more smiles than the parent's face, rocking may not help, smiling is not reciprocated. Parents often feel that their love is not received—that nothing works. Interaction suffers.

When compared with parents of normally developing children or to their interaction with non-autistic siblings, parents of children with autism (and/or developmental delays that affect responsiveness) often speak less, verbalize less, and initiate less play with their children (Hastings et al 2005, Rogers & Williams 2006, Siller & Sigman 2002, Sussman 1999). It is not that these parents love their babies any less or have less desire to interact with their little ones. Often they are immensely dedicated and loving. However, one-sided interaction is not fulfilling. We are 'programmed' to respond to interaction, and when our attempts are not reciprocated something in the cycle gets disrupted. We feel misunderstood and may initiate less.

Awareness of how lack of reciprocity can affect communication is why early intervention with families of autistic children often includes addressing dyad dynamics (Sussman 1999). Parents are educated (and validated) about possible reactions and are given tools to help minimize communication failure by looking for signs of reciprocity and proactively maintaining interaction even if the child seems to 'not care.' Therapies model daily interactive opportunities and target development of flexible routines, dyads, and verbalizations (Siller & Sigman 2008). Similar interventions and tools are often relevant for children whose dyadic development was stalled due to other disabilities, trauma, neglect, or abuse (Yehuda 2004, 2005, 2011, Yoder & Warren 2002). Basic interactive dyads form the baseline for communication and must be addressed because reciprocity builds regulation and attachment that then allows the child to free up energies for development, language, and socialization.

Attachment

Attachment can be viewed as the glue that holds our relationships together. It affects how we see ourselves in relation to others in our lives, as well as how effectively we respond to new people, how we perceive and act on our needs and the needs of others, and how we regulate our reaction to mishaps and challenges (Bowlby 1997, Cozolino 2006, 2014, Gomez 2012, Wallin 2007). It is intricately connected to communication through our interpretation of the validity of our needs and our ability to empathize with others without losing ourselves in the reactions of another.

Attachment forms in infancy and continues to develop throughout life, with early attachment viewed as especially important. The two main styles of attachment described by Mary Ainsworth in the 1960s were secure attachment and insecure attachment. Secure attachment is best attained by children through access to sensitive caregiving. A sensitive caregiver attends to the infant by providing consistent and kind attention that does not overwhelm the baby and helps the baby experience regulating. Securely attached babies are available for communication, play, and exploration; they can attend to new information because they trust the caregiver to provide support if they become distressed or uncomfortable. They attempt more independence through socialization, experimentation, and exploration. Their ability to self-regulate allows them to tolerate the occasional anxiety and distresses of life and feel secure that if distress is too much, they will be helped.

Insecurely attached children, on the other hand, remain occupied with attachment and stress. They may avoid attachment, be ambivalent about it, or experience disorganized attachment, and are not as available for communication, play, and exploration. Babies with an avoidant attachment style seem to not rely on others for comfort. Their caregiver may have been unable to respond to them in a sufficiently sensitive way and the child may not know how to use their caregiver to help downregulate distress. They might seem unaffected by a caregiver's departure from the room and show little fear of strangers.

Babies who have ambivalent attachment may seem simultaneously clingy and angry. They might have a hard time letting comfort in and take a long time to recover from distress. Their caregivers may have been inconsistent—sometimes there, sometimes not—and these children do not trust that comfort will be coming or that it will last. They might get anxious fast and remain that way longer; they might experience fear of strangers, acute separation anxiety, and uncertainty that the adult would return or will be there (physically or psychologically) to comfort them (Giovanni 2004, Lyons-Ruth et al 2009).

Disorganized attachment describes the attachment style of those children who are clearly insecure but do not fit either avoidant or ambivalent attachment (Giovanni 2004, Liotti 2004, Lyons-Ruth et al 2006). Children might develop disorganized attachment if caregivers are alternately intrusive and neglectful, scared or scary. The baby both needs and fears the parent. Locked in a double-bind, babies might shut down (i.e. dissociate) or show opposing reactions: reach to the parent while also turning away, alternately walk toward the parent and collapse dejectedly to the floor (Giovanni 2004, Gomez 2012, Henninghausen & Lyons-Ruth 2007, Kagan 2004).

Attachment development and communication development are intricately intertwined. Sensitive care that helps secure attachment also assists children in putting meaning into sensory perceptions, routines, and contexts. When caregivers ensure that babies avoid overwhelm, children are freed to learn, communicate, and explore. In contrast, children whose caregivers are less able to aid them in managing overwhelm and offer less opportunity for understanding experiences may not be as adept at interpreting their environment. These children have more difficulty comprehending their feelings and regulating their bodies. Anxious and/or numb children do not learn well and have fewer resources available for interaction, communication, and learning.

2 Early Language Development
How Language Shapes Reality and Reality Shapes Communication

Language acquisition is a complex task that fills numerous excellent books. This chapter cannot do real justice to the process, but will attempt to offer an overview of some of the main tasks children face and how they can relate to communication through the lens of this book.

To learn language, babies process information without an existing framework and while simultaneously attending to a multitude of other developmental and relational tasks. It is a 'learn as you go,' where nothing has been learned before. A child not only learns the word "bottle," he learns that a bottle exists, what a bottle is, how it feels, what it looks like, that it remains a bottle regardless of being full or empty, that there are things that look and feel completely different which are also called 'bottle.' Words are usually presented embedded in changing contexts by different speakers at different times. So in order to separate the word 'bottle' within the long strings of sounds of utterances, the child must somehow deconstruct these into 'stand alone' smaller bits—i.e. words—and do so before they know what words even are.

Let us consider a situation when Billy drops his bottle and cries. Billy's dad may say: "Oh, what's wrong, Billy? You lost your bottle? Where did it go? Did you throw your bottle again? Did it fall? . . . Ah! Here it is—the bottle rolled under your crib . . . Here you go, Daddy found your bottle!" Billy learns many things in such an exchange, but suppose we look only at the target word 'bottle': It appears in different places in the sentences, embedded within a long string of sounds that varied each time. Utterances are not separated into words as they are in writing. There is little acoustic separation between words during speech as they flow into each other. Pauses are better represented by commas and periods than by spaces between words. Nonetheless the baby's auditory and linguistic system has to somehow isolate a common denominator in all those utterances and connect this particular string of sounds with 'the thing that my milk comes in' (even before the baby has words for 'thing,' 'milk,' 'my,' or 'in'. . .). That babies manage to make these connections, and most of them do it so well, is nothing short of magical.

It is widely believed that humans are 'primed' with the ability to acquire language, and if given the opportunity to do so, babies will learn language (Baron

1992, Berman 2004, de Boysson-Bardies 1999, Dromi 1987, Gleason & Ratner 2009). Indeed babies learn more than one language simultaneously if they are raised in multilingual homes (Bialystok 2001, Harding & Riley 1986). However, the key to language learning is exposure. No exposure, no language. Quality and quantity matter, too, and if language exposure is poor, the child's language will be poor as well (Berman 2004, Beverly et al 2008, Hough & Kaczmarek 2011).

By the time Billy dropped his bottle and had it retrieved by his father, he would have heard the word in varied contexts and often with the visual cue of the bottle. He likely associated the sound combination (i.e. \'bät-°l\) with comfort, possibly including the bottle's nipple or cap or even the stroller bag pocket where it may be carried. Billy probably associates the sound combination with gurgles in his tummy and with the contentment that follows being fed. The word can bring up the smell of the milk, the safety of his parent's arms cradling him during suckling, the warmth of the fluid, the taste, the calming crooning the parents makes as they burp or rock him to sleep after a meal.

Billy may learn to associate the sound combination with his water-bottle, too, then with pictures of bottles in a book, or a bottle held by another baby at the park. He may look at the item when his parent says the word, and by age 7–9 months can look for it if he hears the word said. Even before Billy says his first word (let alone 'bottle') his comprehension for words and his basic vocabulary would have formed. Vocabulary includes not only the words we say, but also the words we comprehend. Normally developing well-cared-for babies comprehend many lexical items before they begin to talk, and when they do begin to speak, there are far more words they 'know' than words they produce. Even one-year-olds can associate words with things as well as actions, persons, locations, and body states (Baron 1992, Berman 2004, de Boysson-Bardies 1999, Gleason & Ratner 2009).

Lexical items are usually acquired receptively before they are used expressively. However, use of a word does not necessarily indicate that the word is understood fully or without errors about its meaning. Both undergeneralizations and over-generalizations happen as words are acquired (Dromi 1987). A child may call her dog "woofy" but not extend it to other dogs. Toddlers often call all men "Daddy." Even when used correctly, words may only have partial understanding. Children may be taught to say "pardon" if someone else is in their way, but they might not know the word is used as "excuse me" or means "forgiveness." Ambiguous words may be even harder to acquire: Hearing the word "trunk," a child might think you are talking about an elephant and not understand you are referring to the part of a tree or the 'boot' of a car. In all semantic learning, the context a word is used in impacts understanding of it (Berman 2004, de Boysson-Bardies 1999, Gleason & Ratner 2009, Ninio & Snow 1996). A child who hears "happy" in connotation of her birthday party, gifts, and Grandma's visit learns to associate it with the giddy sensation of joy. This is very different from how a maltreated child may comprehend the word if birthdays are a mixture of anticipation and disappointment and if she is told: "Aren't you happy to see so and so" when that person abuses and/or scares her. The maltreated child may well be confused about the actual meaning of 'happy' (more on semantic confusion in maltreatment in Chapter 9).

Stages of Language Development

Language development is nonlinear, with spurts and starts, periods of progress, and periods when outward progress is less visible. Additionally, variations in pace, personality, culture, and temperament affect the language path normally developing children take. Yet the general process and stages are remarkably similar across languages and cultures. The following levels of language development are often used to classify language stage but should be seen as descriptive rather than definitive.

The Preverbal Stage (0–12 Months)

Babies communicate from birth. They respond to facial representations better than they would to objects and develop preference to the faces of their caregivers over those of strangers (Nelson 1987). Even newborns respond favorably to calm and smiling voices and respond less favorably to angry, scared, or sad faces (Halla 1999). Babies show preference to human voices and especially to the voice of their caregiver (Vouloumanos & Werker 2007). They show early signs of language development by discriminating language sounds from nonlanguage sounds, and by gravitating toward the sounds of their caregiver's language (May et al 2011, Nazzi et al 1998).

The term "preverbal" is more descriptive of semantic language use than actual "before language." In reality, babies are deeply involved with language throughout their first year. By a few months old, babies recognize the voices of people familiar to them and begin to respond to repeatedly used words (e.g. their name, "Mommy," "Daddy," "pacifier"). Though born 'open' to learning any language, infants just a few months old already show sensitization to the sounds of the language their caregivers speak (May et al 2011, Nazzi et al 1998). Babies develop a heightened ability to discriminate and produce speech sounds of that language to the exclusion of sounds that are not in that language. Though early babbling is similar in all babies, later babbling of a baby exposed to Mandarin will become acoustically different—and more closely resembling Mandarin intonation, pitch, and speech sounds—than that of a baby exposed to Spanish (de Boysson-Bardies 1999, Nazzi et al 1998).

During the latter part of the first year of life, and as their motor planning and control improves, babies become increasingly vocal, producing sounds and sound combinations as well as alterations in pitch and affect. They begin to put together sounds that approximate some of the words they are exposed to (e.g. /baba/ for "bottle" or /mmmo/ for "more"). By their first birthday, babies comprehend many everyday words and expressions, and they respond to—and elicit—requests, comments, exclamations, warnings, and denials (Gleason & Ratner 2009). They participate in reciprocal games and songs and 'wait their turn' to act on anticipated movements (e.g. "hands up, clap clap clap"). They recognize familiar people, objects, actions, and routines by name and can follow simple directions ("Give the apple to Mommy" or "Where's the teddy?").

Exposure to rich, full sentences and communicatively relevant and child-directed language during the first year is crucial for language development, social development, cognitive development, and emotional development (Baron 1992, Berman 2004, Gleason & Ratner 2009, Halla 1999). The foundation for turn-taking, comprehension, listening, expressing, and communicative success is laid early. In fact, by the time recognizable words show up, normally developing babies achieve a whole lot of language learning: sound mapping, extracting meaning out of sound combinations in varied contexts and voices, comprehending words from everyday routine, generalizing words to pictures and parts-of-whole (recognizing 'dog' even when only the head is showing or a bark is heard), and utilizing different communicative intents (e.g. question, comment, denial, approval).

One-Word Stage (12–18 Months)

As they enter their second year, normally developing babies comprehend language and vocalize needs and reactions. They recognize names of familiar people and objects; initiate and offer responses; can point to objects they want or wish to show someone; communicate refusal, distress, frustration, disgust, joy, engagement, and wish for repetition. They take turns in games and follow active songs (Baron 1992, Berman 2004, Dromi 1987).

Children vary in how many words they may say and how fast they add new words. Most first words relate to the baby's immediate life: important people (e.g. Mommy, Daddy, Nana), important items (e.g. bottle, doggie, pacifier, teddy), familiar and rehearsed sounds (e.g. moo for cow, woof for doggy, shh for sleeping, clucking tongue for horse) and important actions (e.g. no, more, come). What is 'included' under a certain word may not always match the adult version, with children using overgeneralizations (calling all men /dada/) and undergeneralizations ('duck' only being their yellow ducky but not ducks at the park or in picture-books) (Dromi 1987).

During the one-word stage—and especially in the beginning—words tend to be pronounced as one- or two-syllable approximations of the adult version (Baron 1992, Berman 2004, de Boysson-Bardies 1999, Gleason & Ratner 2009,

Ninio & Snow 1996). This makes them understandable to those who know them well (e.g. /baba/ for Grandma Barbara, /pa/ for pacifier, /be/ for Benji the family dog, /gu/ for yogurt), but since most babies communicate with (or through the 'interpretation' of) familiar people, misunderstandings are minimized. They are not eliminated, however. Young toddlers have limited control over speech production, and an initially small repertoire of speech sounds can result in homonyms—words that sound exactly the same but are used for different semantic items (e.g. /nana/ for banana, /nana/ for grandma, and /nana/ for the baby's favorite blanket that she uses for her nap; /ba/ for bottle, bag, balloon, and Barney) (Dromi 1987). These homonyms are another reason why caregivers are often best at understanding the child, as they are familiar with the contexts where an intended meaning may be used. Misunderstandings (and frustration) still happen, and become communicative opportunities for tolerating and managing communication failure.

Limited speech-sound repertoire and one-word utterances highlight the dependence intrinsic to young children: They cannot manage without their caregivers, and they cannot 'use another word' or 'say it differently' if they are misunderstood. This dependence underscores the importance of sensitive caregiving. An adult who wants to understand the baby, who tries to take into account the context, the child's intonation, routines, and body language, increases the likelihood of the baby experiencing communication as successful and rewarding. Even when an exchange fails, sensitive adults can offer validation of the frustration and offer comfort and distraction. Toddlers learn that their words matter and that they can use words to affect the world around them. This helps them feel safe to experiment with new sounds and words. They realize that words have power when adults respond to their communications with caring and affection. Language becomes a way to get their needs met, express their wishes, comment, and engage.

Babies who receive less than sensitive care, however, may be inclined to vocalize less and may experience more frustration and failure when they do. Babies who do not hear much language during caregiving interactions can be less likely to use language to connect. They may not know how. If their experiences were discouraging and they were yelled at for being 'unclear' or 'not knowing what they want,' they may experience speaking as intimidating and curtail their communication attempts. They are less likely to experiment with new words and often receive less encouragement for it.

The one-word stage tends to last from a few weeks to a few months, and by its end, children often label everyday items, names, and actions. They can anticipate events, understand the rudimentary aspects of cause and effect (you keep throwing your toy and Mommy may put it away, you touch the outlet and Mommy says "No!"). They can use intonation to embed intention into their one-word utterances and can change their tone depending on who they are communicating with (Dromi 1987, de Boysson-Bardies 1999, Halla 1999). They comprehend many everyday sentences describing actions, directions, noting, and explanation. They also produce long strings of sounds called "jargon" or "gibberish," where they experiment with modulating their voice in (often hilarious) semi-conversations (Baron 1992, Berman 2004, Gleason & Ratner 2009). Then, one day, they put two words together and language is transformed.

Two-Word Utterances (aka 'Telegraphic Speech') (18–24 Months)

There is a wide variation in the size of toddlers' vocabulary by the time they begin combining. However, the vast majority will have well upward of 50 words and often several times that. Some children exhibit a vocabulary spurt right before combinations arrive, adding new words every day and repeating many words they hear (Dromi 1987, de Boysson-Bardies 1999, Gleason & Ratner 2009, Ninio & Snow 1996).

Early two-word combinations are devoid of 'connecting words' and tend to contain content words, hence the term 'telegraphic speech.' While simplistic grammatically, these two-word combinations are used for conveying complex pragmatic intents. Toddlers express actions ("Daddy come," "Mommy up," "more hat"), cessation ("no more," "all gone," "Daddy work"), possession ("Tommy hat," "Mommy hat"), narration ("Nana come," "Nana bye-bye," "doggy woof"), and many more (Baron 1992, de Boysson-Bardies 1999, Ninio & Snow 1996). They imbue their economical utterances with much purpose and intonation, and usually know exactly what they mean in their combinations. Unfortunately things may not be so clear to the adult. The child may say the same combination (e.g. "Mommy hat") to communicate different things (e.g. This is Mommy's hat; Mommy needs her hat; Mommy help me with my hat; Where is Mommy's hat; I'm wearing Mommy's hat; etc.). These ambiguities, combined with the child's conviction that others must know what she means just because she herself knows it, create ample opportunity for communication failure, frustration, and tantrums.

Sensitive caregivers who are tuned to a child's needs address misunderstandings with patience and empathy. The child might still feel frustrated and upset that the adult 'isn't getting it.' However, she may sense that the adult is truly trying to help, especially when the adult has helped her feel better before. Communication failures and re-tries provide opportunities to learn that others may not always understand what she wants. Working toward mutual understanding helps toddlers learn that they are separate beings and that their reality is not completely shared by another (Ninio & Snow 1996, Halla 1999). If the exchange finally succeeds, the experience of shared delight and relief of being understood reinforces that communication is worth the effort. This motivates the child to work to become increasingly more proficient in communicating.

Communication failures can be harder when children do not have sensitive caregivers and ambiguities become fodder for misunderstanding. Frustration in the adult combines with disappointment and discouragement in the child, especially if the toddler's frustration escalates and punishment follows. For these children, verbal communication may not feel so positive. They might view words as ineffective, frustrating, and potentially scary. They are likely to resort to actions instead of words—pulling, pushing, grabbing, biting, crying—behaviors that often lead to anger, punishment, and more frustration. Repeated unresolved communication failures may lead children to infer that they can exert little influence and that trying to express needs only brings on more upset. They may alternate between passivity and tantrums.

Simple Sentences (24–36 Months)

Normally developing children may use 'telegraphic speech' for just weeks or a few months, but as they complete their second year, toddlers usually begin using simple sentences such as "I want milk" or "Daddy is sleeping." No longer telegraphic (though still simplified), sentences include morphological and grammatical indicators and word-order that approximates that of the language the child hears. Along with the increased complexity and length of toddlers' utterances, vocabulary growth continues rapidly. Children can add new words practically daily and surprise caregivers with words no one knew they had acquired. Two- to three-year-olds enjoy singing songs and acting the movements (e.g. ring-around-the-rosy). They discover the hilarity of saying silly things and delightedly correct other people's errors (e.g. "No, Daddy, Mommy is not eating, Mommy is drinking!").

Toddlers' sentences are simple but comprehension extends to more complex ones as well. They can follow directions such as "go get your coat and put it on so we can go to the park" or "See Daddy's book on the table? Please give it to him." They adore stories, memorize familiar ones, and may stop a parent who 'skipped' a sentence in a favorite book. Children adjust their tone in symbolic play, begin to use language to engage other children in joint play, comment on their and others' actions, and specify choices. They indicate possession, describe cause and effect, tell stories, and bargain, and they may speak untruths to avoid the consequences of a misdeed.

Two-year-olds increasingly use language to communicate and control the environment. They begin to show an ability to regulate their reactions and delay gratification, though they often do so imperfectly (e.g. they may say "it my toy" and reach for the item rather than just grab it from the other child; they may complain to an adult, "Ben push me!"). As part of evolving social sophistication, toddlers intentionally insert social words (e.g. please, thank you) into their sentences to elicit approval and increase the likelihood of getting what they want (Berman 2004, Ninio & Snow 1996, Halla 1999).

Toddlers of that age delight in repetition. They may want the same story every night, the same pajamas, the same food, the same cup, the same video you had to play nine hundred times. Repetition is soothing and toddlers find it reassuring, but it also provides opportunity for practicing things they already know and anchors them in a world where much is going on that the toddler cannot control or do well yet.

Language becomes increasingly satisfying as toddlers gather words to express what they want and to engage others' attention. They may use language to name feelings and the facial expressions and tone of voice that indicate those feelings (e.g. "Mommy is sad," "I am angry!"). Their communication expands to include people outside their immediate daily routines, and their increased intelligibility and approximate use of recognizable sentences help foster successful communication (Berman 2004, Landry et al 2006a). When misunderstandings happen, caregivers often need to step in to clarify them or to comfort a little one who does not quite have the words for what they want.

With continued narration by sensitive caregivers, toddlers make semantic connections between feelings, physical states, and events around them (e.g. "I understand you're angry we can't go to the park, but it is raining and everything will be wet. Maybe we can go later." Or "I'm sorry you feel sad because your truck broke. I know you love that truck a whole lot. Can I give you a hug to comfort you?") (Cozolino 2006). Children whose caregivers are less sensitive may have a harder time making such connections (e.g. if Mommy is angry whether the child is 'good' or not; if Daddy yells at the toddler to shut up even though she is crying because she is overtired) and may use less words and more actions. If asking nicely for a cookie is ignored or your hand is slapped away, you might as well take your chances and try to grab one . . .

Complex Sentences and Morphology (3–5 Years)

Three-year-old children are speaking beings. Some may be shy with strangers but chatter plenty in familiar situations. If raised in a bilingual (or multilingual) home, they usually speak more than one language quite fluently, and address the right person with the right language, transitioning between languages fluidly if with some word mixing (Bialystok 2001, Harding & Riley 1986, Quin Yow & Markman 2011). Their speech is generally intelligible (even if they delete some sound combinations or produce some sound substitutions—e.g. /s/ for /sp/, or /w/ for /r/). They can describe people and places, preferences and dislikes. They can offer input about actions, motives, and feelings (Berman 2004, Gleason & Ratner 2009).

The preschool years are signified by a rapid and constant expansion of social, relational, and cognitive skills, all of which are reflected in and fed by growth in language and communication. The child's speech is intelligible enough for most people to understand (with some allowance for speech-sound immaturity such as lisping), and they can provide basic autobiographical information such as theirs and their parents names, where they live, their likes and dislikes, and sometimes things they should not share. Preschoolers' social awareness is still evolving. They may disclose information (amusingly or embarrassingly) about private or awkward things (e.g. "My daddy has stinky feet," "Mommy said Grandma is a witch," "Do you have a vagina button?," "Why do you have big boobies?").

Between the ages of three and five, children's language grows exponentially. Their vocabulary, understanding, listening skills, memory, cognitive abilities, conceptual abilities, interests, and social skills all evolve in tandem with language rules for narrative, vocabulary, grammar, and pragmatics (the rules for language use) (Berman 2004, Halla 1999, Ninio & Snow 1996). Their ability to internalize their language's rules is quite amazing, and we often see proof of rule acquisition through errors that 'clue' us to the rule they are processing in their amazing little brains. A child who used proper verb inflection may begin saying, "He gived it to me" or "I buyed it"—offering a window to the acquisition of regular past tense in English. Having 'figured it out,' the child applies the rule, and irregular verbs appear wrong because the rule was used on them too (Gleason & Ratner 2009).

Cognition develops right alongside language, and preschoolers often learn concepts and the words for those concepts simultaneously. They learn about color and names for many colors; size concepts and words to describe them (e.g. big, small, medium, largest, smallest, tiny, tall), prepositions (e.g. on, in, between, behind, next to, through), quantity and ordinal sequences (e.g. more, less, zero, all, none, first-second-third-fourth-fifth-last). The world becomes explained and explainable, described and deciphered. Language allows preschoolers to engage, inquire, listen, and question things in the world around them. Children are often fascinated by nature, by how things move, mix, grow, blend, combine, get put together or taken apart. They experiment with any substance they are allowed to touch (and some they are not allowed to, testing boundaries along the way). They learn words for parts-of-wholes (e.g. steering wheel and trunk on a car, wheels and wings on plane), and specific verbs for specific actions (e.g. skiing, sledding, skating; crying, pouting, whining, frowning).

The preschool years are also marked by increased social interest, symbolic play, and elaborate and verbally planned pretend play with other children (especially with peers) (Halla 1999, Mashburn 2008, Ninio & Snow 1996). Normally developing children enjoy listening to stories and feel secure experimenting with how it would feel to play a role. The line between reality and imagination can be blurry, and children may feel worried about what to believe (e.g. get scared of Daddy's "lion act") and need reassurance (e.g. Daddy lowers his 'claw' fingers, and speaks normally) as they become increasingly adept at moving between roles. Role-play can be harder for children who did not have as much opportunity for positive social interaction (let alone if they had negative input, rejection, and maltreatment).

The spectacular development of language during preschool years allows well-developing children to weave stories (and yarns), narrate their experiences, and tell jokes. They begin to understand some everyday expressions and to listen simultaneously to the words and the context they are said in. They discover that "to have a heart of gold" is to be kind, and "raining cats and dogs" means drenching downpours. This process of deciphering symbolic language, metaphor, sarcasm, pun, and idioms begins in preschool but continues throughout childhood and into the teen years (Berman 2004, Gleason & Ratner 2009). It is enriched by exposure to stories and literature (Heymann 2010, Landry et al 2006b, Mashburn et al 2008, Schiefelbusch 1986).

Toward the end of the preschool years, well-cared-for (monolingual as well as bilingual) children in literate societies start attending to written language as something that carries meaning too. They notice rhyming, names and sounds of letters and develop early phonological awareness and prereading skills (Adams 1994, Gleason & Ratner 2009, Landry et al 2006b, Davison et al 2011). Some enterprising children even teach themselves how to read.

Elementary and Middle-School—Continued Progress to Overall Mastery (6–12 Years)

Children usually speak well and can convey many ideas by first grade, but language development continues throughout childhood. Vocabulary continues to grow rapidly in all word categories (e.g. nouns, verbs, adjectives, adverbs), sentence structure becomes more complex, and children become capable of comprehending and using increasingly specific language terms (Berman 2004, Gleason & Ratner 2009). They learn to decipher and use ambiguous language (e.g. homophones, passive language forms) and symbolic language (e.g. metaphors, similes, idioms) (Heymann 2010, Ninio & Snow 1996). Their ability to utilize language to explain the world around them and their inner world increases and children increasingly reflect on theirs and others' thoughts, ideas, perceptions, and motivations. Language becomes a sophisticated tool for connection, communication, social organization, dialogue, bargaining, persuasion, planning, and more.

Language grows in both depth and width throughout the childhood years, with children adding about 3,000 new words annually, to about 40,000–50,000 by the end of high school. Parental input continues to be important, and a significant number of new words come from reading and world-knowledge (Gleason & Ratner 2009). Reading and being read to become highways for language expansion, and because well-cared-for children tend to be read to more often than children who are less fortunate, this can add to disparities in language between well-cared-for and maltreated children (see Parts 3 and 4).

Adolescence—Continued Vocabulary Enlargement and Language Sophistication

Teens are expected to be quite proficient in language use, but communication development does not end in primary school or middle school. Vocabulary continues to expand throughout life and lexical development is enriched by reading, narrative, and dialogue (Nippold 2007). Stories, lore, fables, classic writings, plays, and newspapers involve rarer language items not in everyday oral language and augment one's vocabulary and comprehension. Idioms, puns, sarcasm, and satire are often used in teen literature and communication, and slang expressions are often reflected in teens' oral speech (Berman 2004, Ninio & Snow 1996, Nippold 2007).

Teenagers may seem taciturn and display a proclivity to one-word utterances in response to adults' queries. However, their inner life is often thrumming with words, thoughts, plans, turmoil, and tangled emotions. Little can make adolescence an easy time, but having words for these experiences can make it a little less confusing, so that the teen can at least have the choice to put their experience in words. Some do so through poetry, blogging, and journaling; others through endless conversations (electronic and otherwise) with friends.

Social life is a focus in adolescence, and communication on all its layers (verbal and otherwise, real and imagined, expressed and inferred) becomes of paramount importance. Moral and philosophical concepts, justice and fairness, hierarchies and groupings, right and wrong all get explored through discussion, arguments, debates, and bargaining—all of which require language skills and ability to use and comprehend nuances of expression and communication.

In summary, children vary in the speed of their language development, the scope of their vocabulary, talkativeness, and affinity and interest in conversation. However, all normally developing children follow the same basic steps of language development, if provided with adequate exposure. The quantity, quality, context, and communicative opportunities children are afforded are all integral to the quality and scope of their language acquisition (Baron 1992, Berman 2004, Cozolino 2006, Mashburn 2008, Ninio & Snow 1996, Yoder & Warren 2002). Sensitive, narrating, and reflecting care allows optimal conditions for language development in babies, children, and teens; maltreatment and overwhelm can hinder its unfolding.

3 Socialization, Semantics, Humor, Symbolic Language, and Empathy

Socialization and Communication

We are programmed to connect. When young, we cannot survive without others, yet even as adults most of us seek connection. Forming and maintaining relationships require that we communicate: to let our needs be known, to understand and respond to others' needs, to share our thoughts, plans, and ideas. Human connection is so fundamental that people find ways to communicate even at great odds and in spite of many limitations. It is no wonder that they do, given that humans communicate almost all the time: in words, actions, posture, tone, expression, and more. Even choosing to not communicate is a message. Our relational world is shaped by our socialization, by how we learned to communicate with others overtly and covertly, directly and indirectly, intentionally or not (Bowlby 1997, Cozolino 2006, Gaensbauer 2011, van der Kolk 2014).

Much of everyday human communication is mediated by language, even if not all of it is verbal (e.g. shrugging, smiling, waving, handing a requested item). Language—both verbal and non—allows us to express ourselves and to understand the experiences of others, plan for the future, discuss the past, deliberate, bargain, tell stories, and seek advice (Berman 2004, Halla 1999, Ninio & Snow 1996). Crucial though it is, language is insufficient without communication—pleasant or unpleasant, wanted or unwanted, rewarding or annoying. Not only is our connection to others mediated by language, but also our internal dialogue and experience, our beliefs about the world, others, and ourselves (Cozolino 2014, Siegel 2012, van der Kolk 2014).

Humans have an innate drive to communicate, but the skills and ways to do so socially are learned, and communication is shaped by language, interactions, and experiences. Language enables negotiating, thinking, theorizing, narrating, contemplating, and relating. It is at the base of both social and academic learning (e.g. reading, writing, mathematics). Social and moral concepts are intricately connected to the language with which we describe, define, and understand them. It is language that enables societies to make rules and explain them, as well as object to rules or renegotiate new ones. Language shapes culture, societal roles, and varied interactions. In the reciprocal reality of communication, socialization shapes language and language shapes socialization. What impacts language and communication also impacts perception of self and others, behavior, and how we explain it or understand it in others (Cozolino 2014, Halla 1999, Ninio & Snow 1996, Rogers & Williams 2006, Siegel 2012).

Meaning and Reality—A Reciprocal Bond

Reality is a highly subjective experience. People often use words to share it with others through verbalizing inner experiences and thoughts. The meaning we put into our reality draws deeply on the contexts and narratives that were communicated to us during our earlier (and often earliest) experiences.

Three-month-old Josh cries in his crib. His father enters the room and scoops the infant into his arms. "Hey little buddy," he says gently, patting the infant's back. "What's wrong? Why are you crying? Need a change of diaper?"

He lays the baby on the changing table and unsnaps Josh's sleeper. "Ah! Of course you are uncomfortable," the father states. "You are all wet! I would be crying, too . . . No worries, buddy boy," Josh's dad continues talking as he removes the wet diaper, cleans and dries the baby's skin, and wraps him in a clean diaper. "There you go. A nice dry diaper . . . and your cute teddies pajamas from Nana . . . Let me snap it closed . . . snap, snap, snap . . . All done. I bet you're hungry, too. Let's go find Mommy so she can nurse you."

Josh's very reality is molded by his father's words and actions. His dad's narration teaches him the preliminary meanings of "wet" and "dry," along with "crying" and how it relates to being uncomfortable. He is learning that his bodily sensations have meaning and can be described: "Hungry" connects to the discomfort in his belly and the milk he will soon get to soothe it. Josh listens to the comforting and affectionate cadence of his father's speech. He is learning that his own voice brings caregivers and comfort, that he is precious, that his needs matter, and that he is not alone. He is learning that voice, proximity, and soft touch are how people interact.

What a child experiences becomes his or her reality (Berman 2004, Cozolino 2014, Denham 1998, Ninio & Snow 1996, Schore 2012, Siegel 2012, van der Kolk 2014). If the adult's language and actions offer comfort and calming, the child's reality is that experiences have names and that words can communicate those experiences in ways that others understand and respond to. If reactions to the child do not resolve discomfort or even aggravate it, the child might learn that communication does not work well. They might find words confusing and not know when and how to use them. If an adult laughs at a child's fear, saying: "What are you screaming about? That's not scary, it's funny!", does this mean that feeling scared is funny? Does crying make others laugh?

Confusions happen even with the most sensitive care. A parent may laugh when he sees the infant plop down at the sound of sneezing, but if the child is startled or cries, the parent would comfort her, validate her safety, and apologize for laughing. The existing framework of sensitive care helps repair the confusion. However, if resolution does not happen and if there is no framework of sensitive care to fall back on, confusion remains and can intensify. If when a baby cries the adult responds with: "Shut up already! You are such a pain," the baby may not learn that discomfort has meaning and might struggle to understand satiety, need, or calm. She could find crying scary.

Language shapes our reality, and our perceptions affect our experience and communication. The way we feel shapes how we react, and the words that accompany our experiences become the tools for describing and understanding similar experiences (Baron 1992, Berman 2004). Language helps us talk about what we see, how we understand it, and what we think others want to know (Ninio & Snow 1996). Young children learn how to do this through the rules they learned and internalized from their caregivers (Halla 1999, Landry et al 2006a, Rogers & Williams 2006).

If the rules for communication and meaning at home match the rules of the larger society, then children transfer fairly smoothly into wider social circles. Happy means happy, sad means sad, hungry means you'll get food, crying means you'll get comforted, talking means you'll be listened to, others talking means you need to listen, taking turns means that it will soon be yours. However, if the rules in the microcosm of an early childhood home are incongruent with (or even opposite to) the rules in the wider society, social connection may prove confusing (Beverly et al 2008, Cross 2004, Fox et al 1988, Ninio & Snow 1996, Perry & Szalavitz 2006). Even if preschool, friends' homes, and distant relatives offer a sensitive way of relating, the child may find the change confusing and interpret words and interactions according to what she had internalized (Yehuda 2005, 2011). Children often cannot explain what they misunderstand and so adults may not realize what the child's confusion is about, but glimpses into children's relational dynamics and beliefs during play can offer a mirror to their world (Gomez 2012, Silberg 2013, Wieland 2011).

Symbolic Play—Practice Makes Perfect

Three-year-old Michael loves 'being' fireman. Every container becomes a 'helmet' and every long item a 'hose.' His big brother Sam's jacket is his 'fireman coat' and he runs around the house imitating a siren as he 'puts out fires' everywhere—on the couch, under the bed, in the closet, on the dining table. Nine-year-old Sam gets irritated when his little brother uses his coat and screeches across the living room. Michael's parents acknowledge Sam's annoyance, yet ask him to be patient. "Michael got quite scared when we had the small fire in the kitchen last month. He is working through it in his own way. Being a fireman helps him feel less helpless. Also," the father chuckles fondly, "you had your Superman period . . . ran around in nothing but your Superman underwear and Mom's scarf for a cape . . ."

Play is a hallmark of childhood; a practice of skills to come. All young mammals play, stalk, feint, and mimic adult behaviors, but the symbolic play of young humans also includes increasingly complex communication skills (Konner 2010, Ninio & Snow 1996). Symbolic play allows children to gain mastery over sequence, cause and effect, narrative, role-play, consequence, social rules, empathy, humor, and magical thinking. Early symbolic play emerges when babies 'feed' one of their toys or rock a teddy bear or doll to sleep. From then on and throughout early childhood, play evolves to complex play-schemes with mimicked and invented narratives, characters that shift roles, and a mix of fantasy and reality. Children play house, doctor, teacher and students, cops and robbers. They also play Superman, princess, and scary tigers. Their play can include fairies, magicians, and imaginary friends.

Toddlers initially play side-by-side, watching each other and occasionally cooperating, but by age three, children routinely play with peers, and social play increases in preschool and kindergarten. Preschoolers negotiate roles and the change of roles, plot scenarios, and accommodate new players or changes in context. Even when they play alone, children assign roles to toys and objects and talk to them and 'for them.' Associations and imagination flow: A bed can be a ship, a mansion, a car, a fortress, a magic carpet. A spoon can be a sword, a wand, a trumpet. A stuffed horse can be a baby brother, a stallion, or a stealthy co-conspirator. As part of practicing social roles, preschoolers often experiment with applying the social hierarchies they perceive around them or find in stories and movies. They try on desirable and less desirable roles and alternate being the 'good guys' and 'bad guys.'

Play is essential. We expect children to spend a part of every day in some form of it, and when they do not do so, we worry. It is through symbolic play that social rules are rehearsed, impulses are modulated, boundaries and rationale are negotiated, and language is practiced and expanded (Halla 1999, Ninio & Snow 1996, Yehuda 2011). Symbolic play is serious developmental work. It allows the child to practice concepts and share information with others, as well as negotiate social strata and role-play themes that may be out of reach in the real world. It is also intensely communicative and forms the foundation for friendships and peer relationships throughout life.

Children's reality is reflected in their play: how they perceive and what they expect of others, themselves, and the world. What children do and how they do it; what they don't, won't, or can't do; who they play with and who does not play with them and why are all clues to the internal world of the child (Brinton & Fujiki 1989, Cross 2004, Danon-Boileau 2002, Gomez 2012, Schaefer et al 1991, Silberg 2013, Wieland 2011).

Well-developing children's play is imaginative and often unselfconscious. They practice both serious roles and silly roles, recreating scenarios from books, movies, and the day-to-day. They delight in the unexpected and absurd and insert silliness and experimental jokes into their play. They may dip their toes into guilt and embarrassment, but their play often focuses on joy, success, cooperation, and empathy. Children experiment with aggression and villainy too but monitor their actions and their playmates' reactions carefully because they know that excess roughness will make them less desirable playmates. Other children, especially those with communication and regulation difficulties, may not be as adept at 'reading' their playmates (Ninio & Snow 1996, Rogers & Williams 2006, Silberg 1998). They may be too aggressive, too possessive, or too mean. Both children and adults gravitate toward children who are better attuned and more fun to play with (Blanc et al 2005, Landy & Menna 2001, Schaefer et al 1991), which further limits the social-play opportunities of a socially clumsy child.

Humor and Empathy

Six-month-old Sandy is playing on the floor. She tries to get to her toy. It is beyond her reach but her hand grabs onto something else. She pulls, and the blanket plops onto her head. Surprised and alarmed by the sudden dark, her face contorts to cry.

Then the dark is gone and her mommy's face appears. Her mommy is smiling. "There you are!" she calls playfully. "Peek-a-boo!" She drapes the blanket over her own face. "Where's Mommy?" she calls before removing it, grinning. "Here I am!"

Sandy giggles. The mother covers the baby's head, but this time when it gets dark Sandy is not alarmed but expectant. She laughs when her mommy's face appears and disappears. Peek-a-boo is funny. It makes a laugh.

People laugh. While humans may not be the only living things to appreciate humor, there is no question that laughter is an integral part of every human community and has been so throughout history. Humor can be gentle or cruel, subtle or obtuse. It can address and point out aspects of reality that are difficult or upsetting. It can also make us appreciate the intricacies of ambiguity, puns, expressions, and word play.

Because funny things often highlight oddities or extreme behavior, one must first have an understanding of the expected (Bell et al 1986). Oftentimes when we do not get a joke it is because we do not understand the context sufficiently to recognize the unexpected (Ninio & Snow 1996, Suits et al 2011). Funny can be quite personal—infants can find torn paper or a sneeze hilarious—but even with idiosyncratic silliness, laughter has a reciprocal (and sometimes contagious) element. The baby laughs and the caregiver smiles and repeats the laughter-inducing event. The baby laughs again, and the caregiver laughs in response, repeating the silliness. Funny becomes funnier because it is shared.

Laughter is social. At its best, laughter is a joyful experience of shared delight that reconnects and enhances well-being. At its worst, laughter is a shaming and isolating experience of being laughed at or laughed out of a group. The outward context may be the same, but the communicative intent—or interpretation—is starkly different. What is 'funny' and how it is used and interpreted often depends on earlier experiences with laughter and whether it was used empathically or not.

Just as in children's social play, empathy helps mediate laughter. Preschoolers laugh at aggressive humor (e.g. cartoons), but only as long as they know no one is really getting hurt. School-age children may curb their response to something they find funny if they become aware that laughter would hurt another's feelings (Bell et al 1986, Ninio & Snow 1996, Suits et al 2011). Empathy helps us take the other person's experience into account. It means being able to recognize the other's reality and how our actions are being perceived, as well as be able to regulate our reactions in ways that will preserve the feelings of another (Fonagy & Target 1997, Halla 1999, Rogers & Williams 2006). The capacity for empathy may be innate, but empathic behavior needs exposure to develop. Even the most empathically resilient child requires some modeling of compassion to recognize it and opportunity to express it. Other children, including many traumatized children, may find empathy more difficult to recognize and internalize (Fonagy & Target 1997, Silberg 2013).

Language, cognition, symbolic play, social skills, and empathy all connect to a child's exposure and opportunities; and so it is not surprising that trauma affects communication and socialization. Children can only utilize what skills they have in order to cope with experiences. A child whose interactions taught her suspicion and fear may react very differently to an event than a child who experienced care and comfort. Trauma coping is affected by aspects of the trauma and the child, but also by the relationships the child has to fall back on, his/her understanding of what is taking place, and the reactions to the trauma the child experiences inwardly and in others (Cozolino 2014, Ford & Courtois 2013, Siegel 2012, Silberg 2013, van der Kolk 2014). What is communicated during the trauma and after it (in spoken and unspoken ways), and how it is understood by children, shapes their perceptions of what happened, themselves, others, and the world.

In order to communicate (verbally and otherwise), we must have a way to understand and/or describe experiences. To relate and interact, children must be able to comprehend, process, and respond. They should have ways to put words to their sensations and perceptions, and experience with discourse and exchange of information. They need vocabulary with which to identify feelings, impressions, memories, perceptions, and needs. These are things we cannot assume traumatized children have in the way that nontraumatized children would. Nor can we assume that trauma is not a factor in the clinical profiles of children with communication disorders. Trauma affects communication; not only the child's language about the event itself, but everyday communication as well (Pearce & Pezzot-Pearce 1997, Putnam 1993, Silberg 1998, 2013, Yehuda 2004, 2005, 2011). To help traumatized children and adolescents, we need to understand trauma and its impact on communication so we can recognize where the children are coming from and understand where trauma had taken them.

Part 2

Trauma, Maltreatment, and Developmental Impact

4   Indirect Trauma

Medical, Intrauterine, Environmental, and Societal Trauma

Medical Trauma—When Caring Hurts

The Potential for Trauma in Medical Treatment

Medical care, meant to provide help, is not often thought of in the context of developmental trauma. Nevertheless medical interventions do carry potential for traumatic impact, especially if they involve pain, separations from caregivers, fear (in the child and/or caregiver), invasive procedures, and repeated medical events in chronic conditions, cancer, and injuries that require multiple procedures (Bryant et al 2004, Carlsson et al 2008, Carter 2002, Casey et al 1996, Drew 2007, Gil et al 1991, Johnson & Francis 2005, Kassam-Adams et al 2005, Kazak et al 2006, Liossi 1999, Pillai Riddell et al 2009, Robson et al 2006, Saxe et al 2005, Shaw et al 2006, Simons et al 2003, Varni et al 1996, Winston et al 2002, William et al 2004, Wintgens et al 1997).

The objectives of medical care are to save life, bring relief, and/or improve function. Health personnel go into medicine to help children, not to traumatize them. Parents understand that what paramedics, doctors, nurses, physical therapists, etc. do is for their child's benefit. It is why they allow medical ministrations even if these temporarily hurt or distress the child. Young children, however, often do not understand medical staff motives, the need for physical intrusions, or the consequences of avoiding them. Even children who understand that doctors are generally helpful may struggle to hold that knowledge if they are ill, afraid, feel misled, or see their parents afraid (Bryant et al 2004, Carter 2002, Dell'Api et al 2007, Kuttner 2010, Saxe et al 2005, Schäfer et al 2004, Shaw et al 2006, Winston et al 2002, Ziegler et al 2005).

Emergency care is often frightening. There may be real or perceived sense of threat to life and the integrity of one's body. Patients may be frightened and feel helpless and uncertain. Pain itself can be terrifying, exhausting, and overwhelming. It can make it harder to focus and understand what is going on. Medication side effects can dim awareness, limit processing, and make events feel disconnected and unreal. Others around the patient may be overwhelmed as well, worried for potential loss of life or the witnessing of agony or called to make important decisions about difficult things.

The situation can be even more overwhelming for children. They may be too young to understand what is happening. They can be terrified by bleeding because they may not know that it can be stopped. Preschool children often interpret words literally: They may think that a broken arm would fall off, that having a 'bug' means that they have roaches inside them. A respirator may sound like a monster. They may believe surgery is where the doctor will cut them up like vegetables in a salad. Because children often believe that to say things makes them real, they may be too frightened to articulate their worries, and adults may not realize the extent of or the specifics of the child's terror. Children old enough to comprehend medical interventions may be too sick or injured to do so. Medications can make them feel odd and oxygen masks can feel frightening and isolating. If they try to remove masks to speak and a nurse places it back on, children might believe that they are no longer allowed to talk or that talking will kill them. They may feel angry, confused, helpless, and afraid (Dell'Api et al 2007, Kuttner 2010, Saxe et al 2005, Winston et al 2002).

Medical crises change the rules: Mom and Dad allow others to hurt them. They may leave them with strangers with gloves and hidden faces to do scary things that hurt. If doctors shoo the parents out, the child realizes that parents no longer make the rules—who would protect her now? Rules about private places and one's body being their own suddenly disintegrate, but instead of fighting the people who break those rules, parents go along with what the hurting people do. They may even thank them for what they are doing. Thank them?!

An overwhelming situation can become even more so if the parents themselves are very distraught or indisposed. For a small child to whom parents are omnipotent, this tilts the world on its axis. Scared caregivers may be unavailable to provide comfort or not do so in a familiar way or convincingly enough, adding to the child's confusion and terror. Medical crises in children can contain all the ingredients for trauma: overwhelm, confusion, pain, helplessness, loss, loneliness, fear, and risk of dying (Bryant et al 2004, Carter 2002, Kassam-Adams et al 2005, Kuttner 2010, Robson et al 2006, Saxe et al 2005, Schäfer et al 2004, Winston et al 2002).

Unlike accidents, which many people agree can be terrifying, chronic illness and conditions that require repeated interventions tend to be seen as something children "get used to." Some indeed do, but for many the overwhelming aspects of medical care are not necessarily relieved by familiarity. In fact this very familiarity can increase anticipatory anxiety and replay previous stress, making subsequent care increasingly overwhelming (Kuttner 2010). Even more so if sick children believe that their predicament is somehow their fault or they deserve it (e.g. when adults say things like "it is for your own good"). Lack of visible fear should not always be interpreted as dissipation of distress. Children may try very hard to be "good"—not cry, fuss, or struggle—if this reduces their parents' distress. They may numb themselves to what is happening, pretend it is not happening to them or is not real, or do whatever they must do to manage (Carlsson et al 2008, Casey et al 1996, Diseth 2006, Drew 2007, Fuemmeler et al 2002, Gil et al 1991, Johnson & Francis 2005, Liossi 1999, Mikkelsson et al 1997, Speechley & Noh 1992, Varni et al 1996).

The Prevalence and Scope of Potential Medical Trauma

Situations that may result in medical trauma are anything but rare. Each year, one in four children in the United States receive treatment for an injury (Kazak et al 2006) and about 2% of children suffer migraines (Stafstrom et al 2002). Data from 2012 report that 3% of babies born alive had birth defects and that 8% of newborns stayed at the neonatal intensive care unit (NICU) more than six days (US Department of Health 2013b). It is estimated that one of every 640 young adults is a survivor of childhood cancer (Drew 2007), with new cancers being diagnosed in thousands of children each year. Based on data from the Organ Procurement and Transplantation Network, about a thousand children a year receive transplants, with more children awaiting one (http://optn.transplant.hrsa.gov), many of whom require ongoing and often invasive treatments. About 15–20% of children suffer chronic pain, and one third of children manage chronic conditions, which may require medical interventions (Kuttner 2010, Newacheck & Taylor 1992).

While not all medical interventions have equal traumatizing potential, and not all children are vulnerable to medical stress in the same way, some types of medical interventions have high risk for trauma. These include: cardiac emergencies and surgeries, burns (painful scrubbing, grafts, dressing changes, surgeries, physical therapy, constriction, disfiguration), orthopedic injuries (restricted mobility, surgeries, painful physical therapy), asthma (40–50% of children suffering from asthma meet criteria for anxiety), cancer and bone marrow transplants, growth deficiencies, dental and facial abnormalities, congenital illnesses (e.g. osteogenesis imperfecta, cystic fibrosis, sickle cell anemia), transplantation, and ongoing life-sustaining treatment. Chronic conditions as well as 'one-time events' might be traumatizing to a young child, and even one-time events can require repeated medical care (e.g. burns, car-accident injuries).

Aspects of Medical Care that Can Be Especially Traumatizing

Young age increases risk for trauma, and the younger the child is at the time of the medical trauma, the higher the risk for overwhelm (Cozolino 2006, Doesburg et al 2013, Gaensbauer 2002, Siegel 2012, Simons et al 2003, van der Kolk 2014). Young children often find it difficult to differentiate the trauma itself from the medical treatment that followed it. The (understandable) overwhelm of parents can further terrify the child, as can the parents' "participation" in causing pain (e.g. a parent applying pressure to an injury or restraining the child fearing a spine injury) and their allowing others to cause the child pain (Diseth 2006, Wintgens et al 1997).

Other risk factors include prior exposure to trauma and stress, behavioral or emotional problems (can make regulation difficult, reduce tolerance for stress, and increase risk for restraining the child), multiple traumatic elements (e.g. injured parent too), witnessing intense fear in caregivers, separation from the caregiver during the event or the medical treatment, high level of pain, insensitive medical staff, and a sense of social isolation or lack of positive support. Developmental delays that make processing difficult also increase trauma risk, as do attachment challenges which make it hard for the child to use the adults to help regulate distress (Doesburg et al 2013, Fuemmeler et al 2002, Koomen & Hoeksma 1993, Newacheck & Taylor 1992, Ødegård 2005).

Medical intervention can traumatize parents, too. Caregivers may be terrified by the possible loss of their child and feel helpless to alleviate the child's pain and terror. The illness or injury and what it entails may feel overwhelming and parents might experience clinicians as rushed, insensitive, or controlling (Bryant et al 2004, Carter 2002, Maciver et al 2010, Shaw et al 2006). They may be terrified if the staff expresses (or is interpreted as expressing) lack of hope or care. Parents may also feel enraged at the circumstances that led to the medical crisis and be (rightfully or not) furious with each other, others, or even with the child. Parental overwhelm can increase the child's anxiety in a feedback loop of mutual distress.

Lack of preparation can make even planned procedures feel terrifying to a child who does not know (or did not understand) what to expect. Both caregivers and health personnel may minimize procedures or not mention them ahead of time, believing that the child does not need to know or worrying about resistance and 'lack of cooperation.' Some parents are told that the child would "forget it anyway." Lack of preparation and understanding combined with the alarming medical setting can cause overwhelm and distrust.

Children's Response to Overwhelm

Lacking the ability to remove themselves from an overwhelming situation, children often dissociate instead. Symptoms experienced by children during and following medical trauma include numbing of sensation and feelings, derealization (feeling like the world around them is not real), depersonalization (feeling like they are not real), dissociative amnesia (not remembering what happened), and shifts in ego states (i.e. feeling it happen to 'someone else') (Carlsson et al 2008, Drew 2007, Kuttner 2010, Saxe et al 2005, Schäfer et al 2004).

Dissociation may lead to children's distress being missed. Some children who "become good" and submit to medical ministrations may have dissociated after realizing that fighting is futile. Some feel guilty about causing distress to their parents and may push away their own distress in attempts to regulate their parents' distress (Carlsson et al 2008, Drew 2007). Young children may believe that if they pretend that nothing is happening, everything would be the way it was before—'making it not happen' may be the only thing a child feels she can do.

Children may continue to dissociate after the medical intervention itself is over, but because posttraumatic responses present differently in children than in adults, their reactions may be missed or misinterpreted. Children tend to have flashbacks that are less episodic and more somatic (Gaensbauer 2002). Also, where adults (and adolescents) with posttraumatic stress disorder (PTSD) may suffer a sense of foreshortened future, young children's very concept of future has yet to evolve and they tend to show more cognitive-perceptual distortions (omens, guilt) (Silva 2004). Traumatized children may suffer feelings of estrangement and can present with changes to imagination, fantasy, and symbolic expression, be less available for play, and become more rigid (Silberg 1998, 2013). Their self-image and self-esteem may suffer too, especially when facing chronic illness, disfigurement, and disability (Carlsson et al 2008, Drew 2007).

Medical Trauma and Attachment Disruption

Secure attachment to sensitive caregivers is protective, but even good attachment can be disrupted by medical interventions (Koomen & Hoeksma 1993, Ødegård 2005). Disruption may happen if children are so overwhelmed that they cannot make use of the parent's care. If children continue to dissociate at trauma reminders, attachment difficulties can persist. Disruption can take place if the parent is physically or psychologically unavailable (e.g. parent is also injured), as well as if the parent becomes part of the trauma (e.g. restrain or administer intrusive treatment to the child). Children may not know how to integrate their need for the parent and their rage at the parent for the betrayal: How can they trust the parent to comfort them when this parent causes pain and fear (possibly the very pain and fear the child needs comforting from)?

The belief used to be that it was best for the child if the parent—whom the child 'knows and trusts'—administered intrusive procedures (e.g. restrained the child, administered home treatments of dressing changes, stretched the anal sphincter). Increased awareness of the realities of attachment disruption is leading more pediatric professionals to recommend that someone else administer treatment (e.g. a visiting nurse), to help preserve attachment (Diseth 2006). Similarly, until not too long ago, parents were discouraged (or outright forbidden) from staying with their hospitalized children (Koomen & Hoeksma

1993). It was believed that children were more cooperative without their parents around (i.e. likely numb and dissociated). Whether for tonsillectomy and appendectomy or following serious accidents, children only saw their parents during visiting hours. For some—especially the very young—the separation itself was traumatizing.

When Mary was three, she was hospitalized for surgery on her urethra. Her parents believed she was "too young and would not understand anyway," and so did not prepare her for the procedure. She was separated from them at the hospital without explanation. In her memory, terrible people did painful things to her privates and no one told her why. Too young to have a concept of time, she thought the hurting things would never stop. She felt helpless and terrified. She could not even see what they were doing. If she cried or struggled, she was simply held down by more "white people" (i.e. in scrubs and caps) and admonished that her "fussing was making it take longer." When her parents finally came, they smiled and petted her and spoke about her "needing to rest and get her strength" and how she "must be good for the nurses who were making her better." Mary was confused—the nurses didn't make her feel better—they made it hurt. She needed her parents to comfort her and was also furious at them for leaving her with the nurses. When she cried, her mother got upset and left the room and then her father left, too. Mary believed they did not take her home because she cried. She did not cry again when her parents visited. She tried very hard to be good, and believed that being good was why she was finally taken home, but something in her broke: She realized she could not rely on her parents for help. Not when it really mattered.

Once home, the hospitalization was not discussed. It involved "privates," and so could not be talked about outside the house either. It was as if the whole thing did not happen. Mary thought maybe it was a bad dream and didn't bring it up. She just became numb and sometimes felt unreal or like she was "looking at everything from outside." The numbness continued and teachers complained she was a "space cadet" and should pay better attention. Her parents chastised her for daydreaming and forgetfulness.

Reducing Risk for Medical Trauma

Medical treatment cannot always be preventable or negotiable, yet there are ways to reduce the risk for traumatization even in difficult medical circumstances. Allowing parental presence can lower anxiety in the child, as can offering distraction, breathing exercises, and possibly medications. Effective pain management and age-appropriate explanations are also important, as is allowing choice whenever possible (e.g. which bandage, who would carry them into the operating room, whether to first 'examine' the teddy bear). Reducing parental anxiety by keeping parents informed and calm improves regulation and preserves attachment in parent and child (Kuttner 2010, Wintgens et al 1997).

There is increasing awareness of the importance of psychoeducation, training, and screening protocols for pediatric medical traumatic stress (PMTS) across conditions and ages (Kazak et al 2006). Identifying and predicting PMTS—including detecting families and patients at high risk—can help with assessment and intervention. Increasing awareness among medical personnel is crucial (Carbajal et al 2008, Pillai Riddell et al 2009, Simons et al 2003, William et al 2004, WHO 2013, Ziegler et al 2005), including educating about how the subjective experience rather than objective measures of disease or injury is important to psychological outcomes.

Where medical trauma has occurred, therapeutic interventions can assist children with exploring their experience and the meaning through drawing, play, dramatization, metaphor, and art. Cognitive Behavioral Therapy (CBT), relaxation therapies, pet therapies, and pharmacotherapy can also help. Individual psychotherapy and family therapy can address the traumatic experience, attachment disruptions, and family dynamics. Group psychotherapy can reduce estrangement and isolation (Kazak et al 2006, Wintgens et al 1997).

An individual child's experience is more indicative of trauma than a particular medical issue (Kazak et al 2006). However, some medical and environmental histories can be especially relevant to developmental trauma and its host of communication and regulation issues. The remainder of this chapter will explore some such histories and the ways they can impact children's perceptions, communication, and regulation.

Medical Trauma: Prematurity

Prematurity carries high risk for medical and developmental complications. Among those risks are motor impairments (e.g. cerebral palsy), sensory impairments (e.g. hearing and vision issues), cognitive and language delays, learning disabilities, neurobehavioral problems (e.g. difficulties with regulation, attention issues), and social/relational complications. These issues are largely attributed to premature nervous system difficulties (Doesburg et al 2013). In addition, the realities involved with premature birth (e.g. NICU) increase risk for overwhelm and its developmental aftermath (Browne 2003, Carbajal et al 2008, Simons et al 2003). Light and noise in the NICU can disrupt normal hormonal and diurnal cycles, and the sounds of machines (respirator, beeping) may mask caregivers' comforting voices. Babies' movements can be restricted, and pain from medical procedures (suction, heel lance) produces physiological and behavioral disorganization that can sensitize the baby to future pain (Simons et al 2003). Rocking and holding normally help newborns regulate arousal, but premature babies have less opportunity for these attachment interactions. The disruptions come at a time when sensory input is the main avenue for laying down neuronal pathways and developing attachment and can affect behavioral and physiological organization and regulation (Anand & Hickey 1987, Browne 2003, Gaensbauer 2002, Kuttner 2010). Premature babies must manage intrusive procedures and overwhelming conditions with nervous systems that are not yet ready for outside stimulation, and without the close contact that follows healthy full-term births. The most vulnerable babies (i.e. low birth weight and early gestational age) face the most invasive medical procedures, least access to comfort, and a higher risk for sensitized nervous systems (Browne 2003, Carbajal et al 2008, Doesburg et al 2013).

Parents of premature babies often feel overwhelmed too (Shaw et al 2006). Scared for their babies, they may feel helpless as they allow medical personnel to stick needles and tubes into their little one. Some face grief and disappointment over the too-early birth and the shattered dreams of perfect birth and healthy baby. In addition to worry about a frail newborn, there may be worry about medical expenses, missed work, household issues, and attending to other children. Some parents are terrified to touch such a very fragile baby. They may feel disoriented by the NICU environment and how not all babies survive. Overwhelmed parents are less available for supporting the baby, and those of especially sick babies may even be advised to "not become too attached."

Attention to newborn overwhelm has progressed immensely in the last few decades. From believing that newborns feel no pain and operating on babies without anesthesia, there is now clear understanding that newborns not only feel pain but are less able to regulate it and can become highly sensitized to pain if it is not properly treated (Anand & Hickey 1987, Simons et al 2003). Improved assessments for (and treatment of) pediatric pain is an active area of research (Carbajal et al 2008, WHO 2013). Eye-masks and noise-canceling earphones help lower sensory overload, and family-centered care and skin-to-skin contact help parents be more involved and available for attachment. Parental calm and comforting reduces infants' distress and pain presentation and shortens recovery from pain reactions (Kuttner 2010, Liossi 1999, Robson et al 2006). This is especially important for premature babies, who endure more procedures than the average newborn and do so with immature nervous systems that are less able to regulate and are at risk for pain sensitization (Browne 2003).

Overwhelmed premature babies might use dissociation by spacing out, staring, and freezing (i.e. sudden stop of crying) (Browne 2003, Gaensbauer 2002, Kuttner 2010), and their sensitized sensory systems can become distressed even by normative stimuli. Many prematurely born children who are raised in attentive homes outgrow their early coping, but some remain hypersensitive. Exposure to additional stress and/or trauma (by maltreatment or overwhelming life situations) raises their risk for continued dissociative coping.

"At the Drop of a Hat"—Serena: Prematurity and Dissociative Sleepiness

Serena was born very prematurely weighing two and a half pounds. She spent three months in the NICU, was resuscitated twice, and was often too frail or sick to be held. "*More tubes than baby,*" *her father told me,* "*and one alarm or other was always beeping. I was scared to touch her and disconnect something.*" *At eighteen months, Serena was brought to me with oral-motor and feeding issues with possible communication delay. She would also inexplicably fall asleep at loud sounds. Imaging and neurology assessment found nothing wrong.*

Noise is not rare in New York City. The little girl was toddling in my office when sirens blared, startling us all. The child's reaction was dramatic. She froze, head cocked toward the sound, and wilted slowly to the floor, closing her eyes. Serena's mother picked her daughter up to cradle her and after a couple of minutes the toddler opened her eyes and wiggled down to play. "*She always did that,*" *the mother said,* "*it just shows more now that she's walking. She did that already in the NICU. Nurses joked she was a most considerate baby—when all the babies needed urgent care, Serena would fall asleep till things quieted down.*" *Joking aside, the baby had been tested thoroughly, but all tests came back negative and the neurologist's view was that* "*premature babies need more time for their system to get calibrated. Some are screamers. This one's a sleeper.*" *One of the older NICU nurses concurred—she'd seen that before and believed babies do that to cope.* "*They find a way,*" *the nurse had said.* "*When there's too much of this noisy painful world of ours, they turn themselves off and fall asleep at the drop of a hat.*"

Premature babies are not the only ones to put themselves to sleep to cope. Arriving to a house following a domestic violence call, a Child Protective Service (CPS) worker I knew found broken furniture, holes in the walls, screaming inebriated adults, and children who not only "slept through it all" but remained sleepy through the loud protestations of the parents while CPS took them away. The children were so "gone" that they were tested for drugs, but none were found and the CPS worker believed the children were "using sleep to escape."

Shut-down sleepiness under a stressful situation can be seen in children adopted from orphanages and following pervasive neglect. An adoptive couple's nine-month-old boy slept through the adoption transfer in an eastern European country and much of the following days. He was difficult to rouse and the adoptive parents worried he was ill. The international adoption agent shrugged it off cheerfully. "Some babies do that until they get used to you. It's much better than baby crying all the time."

"Half-Baked Brain"—Timothy: Sensitivity and Overwhelm

Timothy was born at twenty-eight weeks weighing below three pounds. His father described him as a "*tiny pink wrinkled hairy porcupine, with tubes and wires stuck into and onto everything.*" *Timothy suffered a collapsed lung and underwent surgery to correct obstruction in his intestines, remaining in the NICU for eleven weeks, requiring many therapies thereafter to catch up. A first child, Timothy was doted on by both parents. Angelic looking, Timothy had a smile that could melt glaciers. He also cried and fussed through hours of cradling, miles of walking-with, and inexhaustible patience. He grew slowly, struggled tolerating solids, and caught repeated colds. He hardly babbled and did not talk.*

Timothy was two when I first saw him. Still small but on a reasonable growth curve, he had reached most gross-motor goals but had language delay and dyspraxia (difficulty with motor planning for feeding and speaking). He used a handful of mostly unintelligible sounds and was hypersensitive to textures, flavors, tempera-ture, and touch. He did not like new things or new actions and got overwhelmed easily, stopped responding or shook, whined, and collapsed onto his parents, unable to maintain muscle tone. Timothy's mother could not tolerate him experiencing any discomfort. His father straddled pride and disappointment, and tended to push his son a bit too hard, preferring to forget how frail Timothy had been and wishing him to prove he outgrew it by "being tougher."

Work with Timothy involved desensitization of his face and mouth, along with vocalization, verbalization, and general communication. He cooperated wonder-fully in sessions and made steady progress, but carryover was tricky. Timothy would shut down for home practice as his father demanded too much and his mom too little. The family's various ways of coping with distress reinforced a feedback loop.

A turning point came about four months into our work, after Timothy's father took him to an ice hockey game and they had to leave at halftime. Timothy had clung to his father the whole time, eyes tightly shut, shaking like a leaf. "At first I was angry," the father told me in session the next day. "Other kids weren't behav-ing like their parents were torturing them . . . then I realized they had different beginnings . . ." his voice caught. "I apologized to him when we left. Didn't I, Timo-thy?" He petted his son's flaxen hair. "He wasn't being difficult . . . he was trying to manage . . . I kept thinking about something a NICU doctor said: 'Preemies don't get enough time in the oven, they are managing the best they can with half-baked brains.'"

Medical Trauma: Invasive Medical Procedures

Parents may not know how to explain medical procedures to children, and har-ried medical personnel can have little time (or skills) to do so. It can be tricky to not overwhelm the child with too much information or provide so little infor-mation that the child feels confused and afraid (Carter 2002, Kazak et al 2006, Shiminski-Maher 1993). While a ten-year-old should be more involved than a two-year-old, even young children should not be left in the dark about what is happening to their bodies (Kuttner 2010, Robson et al 2006). Generally speaking, it is best to use contexts the child can understand, to allow some time to process the upcoming procedure, to be truthful (though not overtly graphic) and to encourage the child's questions. Young children can benefit from role-playing the basics of the procedure (e.g. on a stuffed animal) as an opportunity to pre-pare for it and clarify misconceptions.

"You'd Think Someone Is Cutting Her Up Alive . . ."—Abby:
Underrecognized Pain

Abby, age six, was referred to me for "slurry speech," sound substitutions and dele-
tions, nasal voice, and overall unintelligibility. She also had "concentration issues,"
"comprehension issues," and "memory problems," where she "forgot" things she
knew or even what she did earlier in the day. Quite upsetting to the parents was the
"problems with boogers"—Abby did not notice when her nose ran but did not allow
others to touch her face. As an infant, Abby had low muscle tone, which affected
feeding with frequent aspiration. She had repeated ear infections, including mas-
toiditis (infection in the bone behind the ear) at age three which required surgery. At
age four, she had tonsillectomy and adenoidectomy followed by another procedure to
repair adhesions, which required nasopharyngeal scoping and other tests.

Abby began weekly speech therapy with me. Though initially wary, Abby realized that nothing I did hurt (there were areas in her face she said "hurted" and
did not want me to touch) or was more than she could tolerate. She cooperated
well in sessions and within a mere few weeks made improvements in motor function, resonance, and sound production. There was no such cooperation at home,
and "Na'ama work" became a battleground where Abby "pretended not to listen"
when her mother called her to come and practice. On her part, the mother "kept
forgetting" only to demand Abby do more than I had asked "to make up for forgetting," which Abby resented. It also became evident that Abby completely refused oral
hygiene care. The father "stayed out of all this medical stuff" and the mother was
frustrated. "She's an angel for you," she complained to me, "does anything you ask.
At home you'd think someone is cutting her up alive when all I'm doing is brushing
her teeth or even her hair!"

I arranged a parent meeting to move past this impasse, and other issues became
clearer. Abby's parents rarely told her about upcoming medical appointments (or
procedures) to "avoid the inevitable fuss." Paradoxically, Abby would be present during discussions of "future procedures." Her parents believed it was "all over her head
anyway." When Abby "made scenes" during appointments, her father would leave
the room and the mother had to restrain Abby for doctors' examinations. Feeling
guilty, she would later buy Abby presents and need to know that Abby was "okay
with what happened." Discussing it, the parents realized how their conflict and distress played into the problem.

Both at school and at home, Abby "checked out" and had meltdowns when she
received a "consequence" for not listening. Her hearing needed to be monitored, but
it hadn't been tested fully because Abby refused the earphones or the bone-conductor
probe, complaining of pain behind her ear. She also complained about sensitivity in
her mouth but the ear, nose, and throat specialist reassured the parents that "everything looks healed." He noted that Abby was "on the dramatic side" and advised the
parents to "reassure Abby it doesn't hurt."

The next time I saw Abby, I asked about her experience at the doctor. After making sure I was not intending on producing one to examine her, Abby told me that she was "mad" with her mom for holding her down and "tricking her" about going to the doctor. Abby was unable to have fun anyplace, never knowing if the next stop was the doctor, and so felt anxious until they returned home. She was confused about her body's boundaries and her rights to it: Her mom told her about "saying no" but she wondered if that was "just a trick" because her mom and doctors did things even if she said no. Her pain confused and scared her, too. "When Mommy brushes my teeth it choking me," she told me, adding, "and my ear feels burning." Abby hated hair care, but the long golden locks were her mother's pride and joy, and hair care was nonnegotiable, tears or not. "It hurts lots [she pointed behind her left ear], but maybe it doesn't, so maybe I'm just lying. Sometimes it burns and burns and then I make it numb . . ."

Abby's parents listened when I recommended Abby be seen by a neurologist and pain specialist and she was diagnosed with neuralgia and allodynia in her head and mouth. The diagnosis itself helped Abby feel validated and lessened her acting out. Her parents' apology helped even more. Abby was taught visualizations to help manage the pain, and a topical anesthetic helped reduce sensitivity behind her ear. She got a haircut . . . an adorable pixie cut she loved and that allowed her to care for her own hair. She was also made responsible for her own oral care, and beamed when the dentist praised how well she did it.

As part of care, Abby's parents began counseling. Her father got more involved, understanding how his intolerance of medical stuff sent mixed messages to his daughter. Abby was given age-appropriate decisions—who to take her to an appointment or whether to do something fun before or after. In her work with me, Abby's stories of the 'yucky doctor stuff' and 'brave teeth brushing' became material for speech-production practice (more about processing via stories in Chapter 15). Abby did remarkably well. The sensitivity in her left ear ruled out amplification, but simple class modifications helped significantly. Abby no longer 'checked out,' and her memory, concentration, and listening issues progressed dramatically. The sensitivity in her mouth normalized and her intelligibility improved.

Chronic Pain

Abby had endured invasive procedures and suffered chronic pain. Chronic pain is known to have social, developmental, physical, emotional, and cognitive impacts and can have serious consequences: hopelessness, depression, withdrawal from activities and interactions, anxiety, distrust, and dissociation (Kuttner 2010, Liossi 1999, Mikkelsson et al 1997, Varni et al 1996). These can be compounded in children who do not understand their pain, think it will never go away, or believe it means they are dying (Carlsson et al 2008, Drew 2007). Childhood pain is common and yet pain in children remains frequently undersupported and unacknowledged (Carter 2002, Pillai Riddell et al 2009, Shiminski-Maher 1993, William et al 2004). This is in part because of outdated beliefs about children's pain and in part because pain is complex and subjective (Ziegler et al 2005). Infants and small children cannot self-report pain, so assessing it requires an interpretation of the child's reactions and behaviors by an adult. These 'readings' may be wrong, resulting in undertreated pain and prolonged suffering. In all medical exchanges, good communication is important. Children who are asked about their pain do better (Kuttner 2010), and keeping parents educated and supported can help them recognize and address pain without catastrophizing or avoidance (Gil et al 1991, Kazak et al 2006, Liossi 1999, Stafstrom et al 2002).

Medical Trauma: Childhood Cancer

Children with cancer manage many challenges. Hair loss and changes to their bodies make some children feel alienated and unreal. Taste and smell can feel strange because of side effects of medications and make favorite foods taste odd and no longer comforting. It can be confusing (and insulting) when baldness makes people mistake them for the other sex. Children may feel anxious about who will be on hand and whether medical staff will be gentle or rough. Even after remission, cancer continues to affect children. Some suffer chronic pain. Many become overanxious, phobic of procedures, and wary of body positions that trigger treatment memories. Children after cancer often report existential and social fears. They can be hypervigilant to every symptom as potentially life threatening, and many feel torn between relief and guilt for being alive while others die. Cancer survivors face the possibility of relapse and metastasis, and even regular checkups can trigger worries as well as memories of the diagnosis and what followed. Some children worry about fertility and the risk of cancer in their own children (Carlsson et al 2008, Drew 2007, Fuemmeler et al 2002, Liossi 1999, Speechley & Noh 1992).

Many children do not share their worries with others. They may be anxious that to speak will make fears real, or sense that the topic brings up distress in others. Some feel they are expected to be 'troupers,' especially if staff and parents praise stoic, noncomplaining children, or if their fear is minimized or shamed (e.g. "even babies here get this test, and they don't make a fuss") (Barakat et al 2000, Carlsson et al 2008, Drew 2007). Treatment and medications can affect processing, executive functioning, and concentration and make it harder for children to formulate and express thoughts.

"The Girl Who Learned Not to Ask"—Dana: Cancer

Dana was eleven when she began seeing me for language/learning issues and pro-cessing difficulties. She had two siblings, aged twelve and eight. Her parents were middle-class, caring, and responsible. They provided many background details but hesitated on medical history, stating it was "probably not relevant for speech." Apparently, Dana had kidney cancer at age four and underwent surgery and chemotherapy, but the illness was not talked about now that it was "behind them" as the parents preferred to "not cause Dana anxiety by bringing it up."

Dana was described as a somewhat morose but compliant child who cooperated even when visibly tired. She got "glassy eyed" when there was a lot going on or in medical settings, yet did not protest or speak about distress. She reportedly managed to keep up in elementary school but struggled with the more proactive middle-school demands and some days could not do tasks she had done easily before. Teachers did not know whether her issues were related to language, learning, executive functioning, attention, or processing. She had good general knowledge but difficulty utilizing information for planning, describing causation, and offering solutions. She preferred facts to personal opinions and views. Never defiant, Dana did not ask for clarification when she needed help and rarely questioned others' suggestions. Well liked by peers, Dana had no close friends and little excited her. Heavy-set and not athletically involved, she preferred sedentary activities. This was very different than before the cancer, when Dana had been an active, opinionated, and bubbly preschooler. "Maybe cancer made her quiet," her mother sighed.

It seemed cancer quieted more than just Dana . . . Her siblings were five and one when she fell ill. The parents did their best caring for everyone, but overwhelm was managed more with silence than with fury, and the illness rarely brought up. Though Dana changed, she was not showing evident distress, which made avoiding of the topic easy, and Dana's little brother did not even know she had been sick. Dana's parents worried about her future but did not speak of it, cancer becoming a big elephant to skirt without mentioning.

It was not clear whether Dana was at risk for language/learning issues before the cancer or her difficulties were exacerbated by cancer and overwhelm. However, it was plausible that some of her struggles were related to her history. Dana responded well to treatment, and her teachers applied suggestions for pacing and grounding to lower stress at school (see Chapter 14). Dana's use of affective language improved, as did her solutions and predictions. She began asking for clarification. As Dana's narrating skills improved, she voiced more views and opinions; good as well as sad. She would quietly comment self-derogatorily, "I'm stupid," "I suck at everything," and "I'm too fat." She became moodier at home and shut down frequently.

I recommended counseling, but Dana's parents danced around it. They agreed it was "indeed very important" to support a child who endured a serious illness, but did not follow through on referrals, reassured by her improved academics. Their focus became her weight. They used code phrases like "get moving more" or "a better growth curve," but gentle though they tried to be, Dana was already self-conscious about her body. I pondered whether her weight was hormonally mediated and/or related to her specific cancer, but the parents were like Teflon for questions about Dana's health—they would not (or could not) go there. Wrapped in silence about her history and its impact (past, present, and future), I wonder whether Dana even knew to ask.

Medical Trauma: Congenital Conditions and Chronic Illness

Congenital conditions and chronic illness often require repeated medical interventions and may be the only reality many children with chronic conditions know (Casey et al 1996, Gil et al 1991, Janus & Goldberg 1997, Johnson & Francis 2005, Ødegård 2005). Cerebral palsy, cleft palate, osteogenesis imperfecta, Treacher Collins syndrome, neurofibromatosis, etc., can shape children's perception of themselves, their relationships with others, and how they manage pain, anxiety, and discomfort. Life may revolve around respiratory therapies (e.g. cystic fibrosis), infusions (sickle cell), injections (juvenile rheumatoid arthritis), dialysis (kidney problems), and more. For other children life begins healthy, until accidents (e.g. traumatic brain injuries, burns) bring on chronic conditions, repeated painful procedures and therapies, restricted movement (casts, IVs), and invasive treatments that the child is helpless to stop or control.

Pediatric feeding disorders often co-occur with congenital malformations that involve the head and neck (e.g. cleft palate), metabolic or digestive issues (e.g. cystic fibrosis, celiac, reflux), or problems with muscle tone and coordination (e.g. cerebral palsy, muscular dystrophies, Down syndrome). Children are commonly seen by speech-language pathologists for feeding, oral-motor, and speech therapy. Though rarely considered traumatic per se, feeding can be complicated by medical procedures that include the head, neck, and mouth. Chronic hospitalization and periods of nothing-per-oral (NPO) or medications that reduce appetite or make food taste bad can interfere with hunger and satiety signs. Some conditions make eating and swallowing (and/or digesting) painful and might lead to hypersensitivity, aspirations, vomiting, or choking (Piazza & Carroll Hernandez 2004).

When children associate eating with choking or food with pain, they can continue to refuse and avoid foods even after their mouths heal or muscle coordination improves. This creates tension around what is normally a pleasant and bonding interaction. It also affects normal oral exploration, practice, and oral-motor development, all of which perpetuate the problem (Piazza & Carroll-Hernandez 2004). As with Abby's case earlier, even simple daily interactions like feeding and oral care can become overwhelming and perpetuate habitual dissociation and posttraumatic symptoms.

Breathing disorders such as cystic fibrosis and asthma can be overwhelming (Ødegård 2005). Asthma can cause serious medical crises. Undertreatment (e.g. insufficient control and medication) and environmental risk factors such as roach infestations can result in terrifying flare-ups. The double whammy of stress and asthma rates in inner-city children make it especially important to consider trauma exposure in asthmatic children. Children with chronic asthma have higher PTSD prevalence than non-asthmatic children. Vanderbilt et al (2008) found that 33% of severely asthmatic children were hospitalized at least once a year, and 25% met criteria for PTSD. Seventy-four percent of the children reported experiencing traumatic events, and for half of them the most traumatic was an asthma attack, where some thought they were going to die.

Pain and helplessness are flow-charts to overwhelm and dissociation and can be exacerbated by people (sometimes even the parents) reacting in fear, disgust, grief, apathy, ignoring, avoidance, minimization, and rejection (Carter 2002, Dell'Api et al 2007, Drew 2007, Gil et al 1991, Shiminski-Maher 1993, Varni et al 1996, Winston et al 2002). Children with congenital disorders and chronic illness are at high risk for posttraumatic responses of numbing, shutting down, avoidance, freezing, 'going ragdoll,' panic attacks, hypervigilance, and more.

"The Air Monster"—Martina: Asthma

Third-grader Martina was a walking contradiction. Her immature behavior, noticeable lisp, and breathy high-pitched voice belied her physical appearance; the large nine-year-old had already begun puberty. Martina lived with her mother, grandmother, and two younger siblings in a poorly maintained building that forever had problems with roaches and rats. The family was unable to get better housing, which was particularly problematic for Martina, who had severe asthma. The girl's language-learning delays and articulation issues were compounded by attention and memory difficulties, 'daydreaming,' and irritability.

Everything was a struggle for Martina. She wept at the smallest provocation or distress, and her sobbing often brought on whistling asthma attacks. She was to carry an inhaler at all times but sometimes did not have it, claiming the "medicine run out" and her mother "not get it" (from the pharmacy). Fortunately the nurse had added medication for her, but when gasping for air, it was hard to help Martina, as the child frantically pushed away hands offering inhalers and fought the inhalation mask the nurse offered. Panic only exacerbated her attacks. Martina reportedly spent many nights in the neighborhood emergency room, fighting nurses there as well.

"It choke me," she rasped to me after the teacher called me to calm Martina down enough to take her medicine. "Every day the air monster take my air and I canno breathe." I mused aloud about that 'air monster' and where it lived. "Here," Martina pointed to her chest. "It come from the roaches and it make holes in my air and maybe I be dead."

Intrauterine Exposure to Alcohol, Drugs, and Maternal Stress

Some children come into this world with neurological systems already 'primed' for hypersensitivity. For them, even the usually tolerable can be experienced as intolerable. Moreover, they may have reduced ability to regulate arousal states and modulate stress, which further increase risk for overwhelm. Some causes for neurological vulnerability and development are still a mystery, but many other risks are well known. Exposure to alcohol, for example, leads to fetal alcohol syndrome (FAS) and fetal alcohol exposure (FAE), where the physiological characteristics (e.g. small head circumference, flat oro-nasal groove) are only part of the constellation of symptoms. Children often struggle with attention issues, low birth weight, developmental delays, and difficulties with emotional regulation (Barth et al 2000, Martin & Dombrowski 2008). The risk to these children goes beyond alcohol exposure, because maternal alcohol use during pregnancy often takes place alongside smoking, drugs, malnutrition, and/or maternal nutritional deficiencies following poverty, self-neglect, mental illness, etc. Similar risks are true for 'crack babies' (children born addicted to cocaine) and children with other prenatal substance exposures (Albers et al 2005, Barth et al 2000, Miller 2005).

More often than not, the realities that made the pregnancy developmentally risky continue after the baby is born, increasing risk for traumatization through abuse, neglect, and attachment disruptions. Even under the best circumstances, colicky, cranky, fussy, irritable, and hard-to-soothe babies (as 'crack babies' and babies with FAS/FAE can often be) are at a high risk of maltreatment. "Difficult" babies are more likely to be shaken, ignored, sedated, and hit compared with calmer and "easier" babies. All the more so with caregivers who do not tolerate the baby's needs and reactions. Infants exposed to substances may have neurological difficulties with regulation directly related to teratogenic effects, along with issues relating to having an unavailable and/or abusive caregiver (e.g. alcoholic mother) (Thompson et al 2009). They may suffer from malnutrition and untreated middle ear infections that may complicate developmental and communication delays (Albers et al 2005, Barth et al 2000, Miller 2005).

Even without substance abuse, high maternal stress can impact the developing baby. Babies born to mothers who had PTSD during pregnancy were more likely to be born smaller and show lowered cortisol levels compared with babies born to mothers without PTSD. Low cortisol levels are associated with a vulnerability to posttraumatic stress (Yehuda et al 2005). Abnormal cortisol levels were also found in the babies of pregnant mothers with perceived high stress (Leung et al 2010) and in intergenerational stress (Yehuda et al 2007). Because stress and stress reactivity are multifaceted with chemical, environmental, and interpersonal factors, it is important to explore and address past as well as present stress and posttraumatic coping in both caregivers and children.

"Good Child/Devil Child"—Leila: Bipolar, ADHD, or Hell to Tell?

Leila was a first grader at an inner-city public school. She moved through multiple foster-homes after removal from her mother's custody and had language/learning delay and serious attention issues for which she received twice-weekly speech therapy at school. She also had mercurial mood shifts, memory issues, and difficulties understanding how actions and consequences connected. She lied a lot. Small-statured and serious, Leila glared fiercely and fidgeted constantly, threading her thumb through holes she made in every top she wore. She was prescribed Ritalin for attention-deficit hyperactivity disorder (ADHD). An antipsychotic for "probably bipolar" was added after the foster-mother took the child to the emergency room for "going ballistic."

Leila's mother lost custody due to neglect, substance abuse, and binge drinking that began well before Leila was born. The mother had already lost custody of an older child and there was every reason to assume she drank and drugged during her pregnancy. Leila was suspected to have FAE, which was used to explain her developmental delay and difficulty with attending and regulating. Less noted were the neglect Leila had endured and repeated attachment disruption. The child craved adult attention, pushing her way through other children to be noticed. She behaved immaturely, throwing tantrums in class for small disappointments or perceived injustices. She was routinely in "time-out."

Leila entered first grade just months into her current foster placement, and already her foster-mother admitted her patience was wearing thin. "One minute she is the good child and the next she is the devil kid," she exasperated. "You never know what is going to come outta this child's mouth, if her hands will fly to hug you or smack you." Not only did Leila have a hair trigger, but once distressed she was difficult to soothe. She lashed, spat, pulled her hair, and scratched her face. These self-harming episodes were what landed her in the emergency room. "She gets so angry so fast it would make you dizzy," the foster-mother told me. "Whatever they want to call her: ADHD, bipolar, alcohol syndrome—all I know is that she is hell to tell."

War, Violence, and Refugees

Children around the world are exposed to man-made violence: domestic violence, dangerous neighborhoods, armed conflicts, war, and terrorism. This exposes them to loss, stress, and fears for their lives and the lives of those they rely on. In addition to the trauma caused by witnessing violence, children often have caregivers who are overwhelmed, hurt, scared, and ill and are therefore less available to the child. There can be disruption, fleeing, loss of belongings and community, and the ongoing strain of living as a refugee. Survivors escaping violence often worry about family members left behind and about their own legal status and ability to remain safe. They may be grieving for loved ones who were lost. In the midst of turmoil, many refugees have to manage new language, custom, location, currency, livelihood, education, housing, climate, food, laws, and expectations. Overstressed parents can be less available and roles can be reversed. Children often acquire new languages faster than their parents, turning into translators, mediators, and negotiators on behalf of their parents and becoming responsible for managing adult matters at a very young age.

In some families the transitions are managed healthily, and parental attachment and support are maintained. However, for many others parental overwhelm leads to the children being unable to rely on their parent, fending for themselves, and caring for younger siblings and even for the overwhelmed parent. War and violence traumatize adults, let alone children, who rarely understand the conflicts that bring on the violence or the adults' helplessness to stop it. Confusion and overwhelm disrupt their learning, social interaction, attention, attachment, regulation, and sense of safety (Kia-Keating & Ellis 2007, O'Shea et al 2000, Tufnell 2003).

"Africa Bad"—Daweed—War Refugees: When an Ocean Isn't Wide Enough

Daweed was 5:9 when I saw him in the inner-city kindergarten near his housing project. His family escaped an African country and kept silent about their experiences. Daweed began hearing English in preschool after the family arrived in New York. Small and thin, the boy was exceptionally well groomed, arriving with pressed pants, tucked-in shirt, and clean face. He struggled to acquire English and his parents said he spoke less than his three-and-a-half-year-old brother.

Daweed was compliant, quiet, and very passive. He exhibited little social and symbolic play, and his only friend was Shamdu, whose family was close to Daweed's. Other kids mostly let him be. His teacher, who met him at preschool, thought the boy was "not too bright and spaced-out half the time." Daweed was eligible for both breakfast and lunch at school, but he ate little and complained of stomachaches often. In sessions, Daweed was quiet and respectful, rarely initiating conversation but appearing just on the verge of 'checking out.' One day, another child in the small group referred to himself as "African American." Daweed stilled then said in wide-eyed monotone: "No Africa. Africa bad. Africa they have knife. Cut [he pointed to his throat]. You dead. They [he pretended to shoot]. You dead. . . . Africa bad. My grama . . . they cut no good [he pointed to his pelvis]." The children sat stunned. I murmured some soothing words, offered distraction, and helped Daweed with grounding (see Part 5). It was the only time I ever heard him speak of this, though there were plenty of other times he would withdraw, listening or seeing things I could not and wished he didn't either, especially around yells of anger or mentions of knives or dogs.

No one at school knew what Daweed's family endured. His parents were caring and judiciously respectful to the teachers, but when asked to know more "about Daweed's heritage" the father shook his head firmly. "He from America now," he said. The mother sat quietly, wrapped in head covering, her eyes darting warily. He placed his hand gently on the back of her chair—not touching his wife in public but offering support. To change the mood, I noted that Daweed got along with Shamdu. Both parents smiled at that. "He good boy," the father noted. "Daweed also good boy." They refused counseling for Daweed but wanted him to continue in Speech—"he learn talk good is important," the father pressed. "He learn English good. More English from me." When I asked what language they spoke at home, the father frowned. "Little bit English," he replied, "more English better." He did not want to tell me. What real dangers the family had endured and may still fear, I did not know, but the parents' wariness was palpable. Little wonder that Daweed, too, was afraid: His parents loved him but were barely managing their own terror and overwhelm, still in survival mode.

"He Talk Me"—Carl: The Parent-Child

Carl's family sought political asylum in the US when he was five years old. When I met Carl he was eight years old and in second grade, having repeated kindergarten to hear more English (he had moderate hearing loss too) and for "immaturity." The boy was strikingly beautiful and his clear green eyes regarded you with knifing assessment. Quiet around most adults, Carl was rambunctious and loud around his peers, but moody and brooding when he failed or did not get his way. He could dissolve into tears and be unable to explain why he was crying; or lash out with breathtaking fury. Children respected his strength and gave him space when he began fuming. Mercurial or not, there was one person with whom Carl was almost impossibly patient: his younger brother Martin, a kindergartener. Carl never seemed to lose his temper with Martin. He tied Martin's shoelaces, tucked his shirt in, zipped his jacket, wrapped the scarf securely around the younger child's neck, patted his brother's hair, and carried his bag. Martin submitted to his brother's ministrations; Carl behaved more like a parent than a young child.

Carl had enough English for narrative, but his language organization was poor and he struggled to keep on topic or retell an event. His memory was good, but not his understanding of causation or opinion. He could identify why something was a good idea to do or should not be done, but not why or how it might make someone feel. He spoke little about himself or his feelings and did not share much about what he did after school or over the weekend. Nonetheless, as his narrative improved, it became clear that Carl was his brother's main caretaker. The mother didn't work. She was home most of the time but in some way unavailable (Carl only said she "needed her rest"). The father worked multiple jobs and was rarely home before the boys were asleep. It was Carl who ensured that Martin had dinner, bathed, brushed his teeth, and had clean clothes for school the next day. Carl attended to his own clothing, food, hearing aid, and chores; he translated for his mother in the supermarket and laundry room. Carl also cared for Martin when the younger boy was sick and missed many days of school tending to his brother's frequent colds. Other times Carl was absent because he accompanied his father to government offices. "I tell them what he say," Carl explained, "and I tell him what they say." This eight-year-old far-from-fluent reader pored over documents and forms, trying to translate. *"They have big words,"* he noted to me anxiously, *"but it important I not mess it up. I no want be homeless."*

I saw Carl's father at parent-teacher conferences; a heavy-set man in work clothes, hooded green eyes, and hands rough from working. Carl came too—to translate what the teachers said about him to his father . . . and to translate to the teachers questions his dad had. The awkwardness seemed lost on the boy, who led his father through the school's corridors as if he were the parent and his father the child. The father looked simultaneously proud of his son and embarrassed to need his help. "I no good English," he apologized, smiling a shy and bigger version of Carl's smile. "Is okay," Carl interjected immediately in a soothing tone, patting his father's shoulder. "I know lot of English already." Carl's father nodded and raised his eyes apologetically to me. "Yes, Carl lot of English. He talk me."

Whatever the exact circumstances of Carl's mother's, much of the burden was passed onto Carl's shoulders. The boy was also a support for his father. The eight-year-old did not always understand what was asked of him, but he seemed well aware of the potential gravity if he failed. This strong and compassionate little boy watched over his little brother and kept both of them reasonably well taken care of. The bonds of affection between him and his father were clear, too. However, Carl's stress left him unavailable for learning and leaked through in his bouts of rage, intolerance of failure, and abject misery when he wept. He kept it together most of the time but did not know how to let others help.

5   Maltreatment
Neglect and Abuse

Child maltreatment is a worldwide reality and affects children from all income and socioeconomic backgrounds. As many as one out of every 10 children in the United States experiences one or more forms of physical, sexual, or emotional abuse or neglect, usually by a parent or other caregiver (U.S. Department of Health and Human Services [US-DHHS], 2013a). Statistics consistently show close to 1,000,000 substantiated maltreatment reports annually, in the US alone, numbers which are considered vastly underrepresentative of actual maltreatment numbers. Many children face multiple risk factors for overwhelm: maltreatment, attachment disruptions (e.g. fostering), environmental and health risks (e.g. homelessness, asthma), developmental issues (e.g. learning disability), and insufficient support. Childhood maltreatment causes significant stress in children and poses a serious risk to attachment, development, health, and mental health (e.g. Herman 1997, Levine & Maté 2010, Miller 2005, Schore 2001, Siegel 2012, van der Kolk 2014).

Neglect—Parental Inability, Attachment Disruptions, and Institutionalization

Neglect is the most common of all maltreatment causes and represents four-fifths of maltreatment cases in the United States (US-DHHS 2013a). Neglect includes failure to provide physical, mental, or emotional care that impairs or is in imminent danger of impairing a child as a result of the caregiver's acts, whether deliberate or not. It often occurs along with other risk factors (e.g. parental mental illness) and can lead to delays or impairments in motor, language, regulatory, cognitive, emotional, or behavioral development, as well as in acquisition of social, communication, and academic skills (Miller 2005, Schore 2001, Siegel 2012, van der Kolk 2014, Yehuda 2011). Though mostly reported with younger children, neglect continues throughout childhood (older children tend to hide it). Lack of physical care is an obvious form of neglect; however, emotional care is also profoundly necessary. Even if cared for physically (i.e. basic food, clothing, shelter), children who were not cared for emotionally often failed to thrive and many died (Bowlby 1997). The devastating impact of emotional neglect has been validated by science (Schore 2001, Siegel 2012, van der Kolk 2014). It is still evident in children from institutions and orphanages where attention, connection, language, and affection are scarce (Albers et al 2005, Miller 2005); these children often show continued dissociative behaviors and attachment difficulties (Beverly et al 2008, Silberg 2013, Wieland 2011).

Neglected children may not learn how to identify, name, or regulate body states and emotions (Beverly et al 2008, Hildyard & Wolfe 2002, Schore 2001, Siegel 2012, Silberg 2013, van der Kolk 2014, Yehuda 2005). They can become withdrawn and apathetic to affection or indiscriminately clingy and friendly, vulnerable to disappointment, rejection, and victimization by those who exploit their hunger for connection. Clinginess can be mistaken for quick attaching, but it is rarely a secure attachment; it is driven by anxiety, loss, and yearning (Liotti 2009, Lyons-Ruth et al 2009, Schore 2012, Silberg 2013, Wieland 2011).

Locked in a cycle of reasonable needs and unreasonable expectations, some neglected children become supremely compliant, terrified that a mistake would deprive them of the little care and attention they are getting. When inevitable errors occur, the child's heartbreak may be judged as "making a big deal" and "overreacting." Children who believe the withheld love is their fault can become paralyzed by a need for unrealistic perfection: If only they somehow made no mistakes, didn't eat so much, need so much, or want so much, they would be cared for. Self-blame is reinforced when children see that some children are doted upon (e.g. at school), and the neglected children internalize that the only reason they are not loved is that they do not deserve to be. Neglected children can be desperate for connection but have difficulty reading social situations, ending up with miscommunications that reinforce rejection and failure (Pollak et al 2000, Yehuda 2005). They can become vulnerable to bullies who exploit their need as weakness and repeat the ugly messages the child already tells herself. Even without bullying, difficulty regulating and hypervigilance can make neutral interactions activating to a neglected child. A teacher's distracted hello can become 'proof' of dislike, a peer's bland look interpreted as angry or disinterested. Extreme reactions to minor or perceived brush-offs can lead to real rejection that further reinforces the child's sense of being defective (De Bellis 2005, Nadeau et al 2013, Shields & Cicchetti 1998).

To manage the intolerable pain of neglect, children often dissociate to cope: numb, shut down, make everything unreal or 'happening to someone else' (Silberg 2013, Wieland 2011). Many aspects of neglect trigger overwhelm, including instability and lack of supervision, attention, and guidance. Hunger, cold, and exhaustion lower the threshold for overwhelm further, resulting in children who are less available—physiologically and psychologically—for processing information and utilizing available support (Hildyard & Wolfe 2002, Kendall-Tackett 2002, Schore 2012, Siegel 2012, van der Kolk 2014, Yehuda 2005).

For example, many inner-city schools offer at-risk children breakfast and a hot lunch. It is understood that this food may be all some of those children get. Yet that food does not always get to—and into—the children who most need it. Neglected children in the United States and other developed countries may not look famished. The hunger they experience may not be a hunger that kills, but it still is a hunger that hurts, frightens, slows, deprives, numbs, occupies, and steals attention and ability. However, many neglected children do not confide a lack of food. Some keep it secret to protect their parents and from (sometimes valid) fear that speaking up will result in losing their family. Others do not tell because by keeping quiet about hunger they can pretend it is not happening. Some cannot verbalize what is going on (see Melanie's case in Chapter 15), while some go to great lengths to conceal their hunger even if they do have words for it. Children often feel ashamed (Bennett et al 2010). They may avoid admitting hunger if it would disclose an unspoken problem with a parent who diverts money into drugs, alcohol, or gambling. Even elementary school children know that 'telling' of problems at home can lead to something that might feel worse than hunger: becoming a 'foster-kid.' So they may skip meals and deny, minimize, and trivialize their hunger. Hunger pains may be easier to manage than shame.

"She Not So Mean"—Karin: Hunger in a Foster-Child

It took me a while to realize that Karin was a hungry child. She tended to space out and had significant learning issues, but she was neat, cooperative, and almost too polite. I usually kept a large jar of sourdough pretzels in my office for students who may be hungry during session, no explanation needed. The fourth grader always took a pretzel when other students in her speech group did, though she would claim not being hungry and wrap it in a napkin "for later." As other children sometimes did the same, I thought little of it until I found out that Karin was keeping the snack for her six-year-old sister. 'On paper' the two girls were receiving school breakfast, but in reality their foster-mother was habitually late, so the girls frequently missed it. Karin kept the pretzel to give her sister the next morning so the younger girl would not fast until lunch. Though she could take as many pretzels as she wanted, Karin did not want to take more than others had . . .

Case-workers are often too overextended to follow up on attendance at school breakfast, and teachers often assume an uncomplaining child ate at home. Children may not say anything. Some fear mistreatment or—like Karin—endangering an otherwise relatively safe placement. "It's no matter," Karin pled when I casually asked her about breakfast. "What if they take my baby sister another place? She need me! It's no matter, okay? This foster don't hit me and my sister like the other foster place. She not so mean."

Karin preferred hunger to the possibility of worse placement or separation from her sister. I spoke to the principal, who made discreet inquiries and ensured that one of the cafeteria attendants handed the girls milk or a granola bar no matter how late they arrived. To supplement that I instated a bagged 'pretzel snack for later' for Karin and her group mates (to not single her out) in my office. She ate one herself now that she knew her sister would not go without. Karin's attention improved, she no longer shut down with hunger, and was maybe just a bit less occupied with worry.

Neglect's Aftereffects

Some neglect leaves visible marks: malnourishment, stalled growth, ill-health. Other impacts of neglect are invisible but no less indelible. Without a 'good enough' model for connection and attachment, children may not know how to relate or regulate emotions and body sensations. They may find it difficult to read others' faces or interact. They often face developmental, relational, attention, and learning issues that linger even after good care is established. Support is important but not always available. Some pediatric professionals still misunderstand the impact of childhood adversity, delay care, or minimize its potential to help. While some early deprivation and adversity cannot be undone, brain plasticity along with addressing developmental trauma and regulation can assist children to attain healthier developmental trajectories (Gray 2002, Heller & LaPierre 2012, Ford & Courtois 2013, Levine & Kline 2007, Schore 2012, Siegel 2012, Silberg 2013, van der Kolk 2014, Waters 2005, Wieland 2011).

"She Doesn't Know How to Love"—Annie Lee: Attachment and Communication Disruption in Adoption

Annie Lee was adopted at eighteen months old from an orphanage in rural China. Babies at the orphanage were fed and kept clean but received little interaction from the shorthanded staff. After spending months swaddled in cribs, older infants were restrained for hours on potty benches outdoors for "sun and fresh air." Spaces between babies kept them from pulling each other's hair or poking out eyes but prevented much interaction, and the infants were helpless against the toddlers who wandered around, poking and hitting.

Orphanage diet consisted of spoon-fed mush—effective in getting maximum nutrition into children with least mess—and meant lack of experience with coordination and chewing. At adoption Annie Lee could not eat solids. She did have numerous dental caries: Teeth were rarely brushed and babies were put to bed with a bottle to ensure sleep on a full stomach. Annie Lee vocalized very little and cried rarely. Her adoptive parents found her unsettlingly quiet. When held, she was either like a sack of potatoes or a wriggly worm, unable to comfortably relax in snuggling.

At first Annie Lee's parents were told by their pediatrician that the scarcity of vocalizations and comprehension were expected, as the child was "busy absorbing" and the language delay was probably because of differences between Mandarin and

English. The parents were comforted but not convinced—they felt she was "more detached than absorbing" and did not think she had much Mandarin. Still, the doctor reassured them that the child was "closing physical gaps and cannot also focus on language" (a misconception, as all babies learn language and motor skills concurrently in their first years).

When a full year passed with little communication improvement, the pediatrician's hypothesis changed to suspicion that Annie Lee—by then 2:6—could be autistic. He noted the lack of eye contact, her little interest in human speech, sparse vocalization, and stereotypical behaviors (rocking). A neuro-pediatrician formally diagnosed Annie Lee with autism, but a second opinion was inconclusive. An ear, nose, and throat specialist found fluids in her ear, and a hearing test showed mild conductive hearing loss, but the audiologist was concerned about Annie Lee's poorer than expected attention to speech sounds; the child behaved much 'deafer' than she actually was. It was the audiologist who recommended a speech-language evaluation with me.

At assessment time, Annie Lee was barely verbal, hardly vocal, still refused most solids, and, though she enjoyed manipulating toys, showed little interest in symbolic or social play with me or at home, where the parents videoed some interactions. "It is like she doesn't know how to love," Annie Lee's mother sighed sadly. "Like she is lost and cannot find or feel our love" (more on Annie Lee's treatment in Chapter 16).

Some orphanage children may indeed be autistic. However, institutionalized children also receive an autism diagnosis when their behavior is due to early trauma and neglect. Children may not attach or communicate because they have never learned how; they may fail to associate sounds people make with communication or language because speech sounds were not directed at them and were no more meaningful than background sounds. They may have internalized different ways of relating, such as not initiating speech or avoiding eye contact (Gray 2002). In some children, human voices might evoke intolerable grief, leading them to dissociate in self-protection. Some children learn to guard against connection that means repeated loss (e.g. volunteers who briefly showered the child with attention then disappeared, loss of placements, failed adoptions). Some may not know how to recognize or accept care when it is offered.

Just like Annie Lee, neglected children may not cry much or may cry incessantly regardless of soothing. If crying did not bring help, children may dissociate to numb the inescapable distress. They may not know how to use others' comforting. In fact, unfamiliar handling may feel irritating and disorienting: Babies who spend most their days in cribs may be afraid to be picked up—the vestibular stimulation may be overwhelming and they might feel safer in lonely familiarity than in someone's arms. Rocking by a caregiver can be distressing to children who rock themselves to dissociate. Self-stimulatory and self-soothing behaviors like rocking, head-banging, finger-twirling, hair-pulling, and mouthing on body parts may 'look autistic' but can reflect coping by children who were bereft of being communicated *with*. As such they mirror the child's history more than their communicative potential. The latter should only be assumed after children are offered opportunities to learn what they were never taught, tools for relational reciprocity, and other ways to manage their early experiences (Ford & Courtois 2013, Gomez 2012, Gray 2002, Silberg 2013, Wieland 2011, Yehuda 2005). However they coped, children are not wrong to have learned to do what they could. With gentle small-step teaching, children can learn new ways to communicate, relate, and attach.

The Interplay of Environment, Caregiver Overwhelm, and Neglect

Foster-care

By its very definition, foster-care implies loss and disruption, and often adds its own stresses: disconnection, uncertainty, changed rules, and lack of control. Repeated shuttling between placements can be overwhelming to children, especially if it comes on top of earlier traumatization. Over 80% of children placed in foster-care have histories of maltreatment, and many present with attention-deficit hyperactivity disorder (ADHD), oppositional defiant disorder (ODD), depression, conduct disorder, anxiety disorder, and bipolar disorder (Jamora et al 2009). Health, learning, and social issues are common too (Fox et al 1988, Hildyard & Wolfe 2002, Scherr 2007).

Attachment disruption is intrinsic to foster-care, and unmet needs are common. Children can get moved without warning, with every placement adding new losses and reawakening old ones. Even the worst upbringing may have held some familiarity for the child, and awful parents were still the child's only ones. Though hurtful, angry, or neglectful, for the child the parents may have been a lifeline that was severed and is yearned for. Every loss of placement (due to child's 'issues' or not) rips away another semblance of familiarity, and many foster-children learn not to connect. They snail in and numb out; they reject and act out (Sprang et al 2009, Yehuda 2005, 2011). Some act out to 'bring on' a loss of placement just to have some control over their lives and prove themselves right about what they believe will happen anyway. Psychological and emotional needs can be missed. Children often get removed with only the clothes on their backs, leaving behind favorite toys and transitional objects. They may 'lose' their siblings if they end up in different foster-homes. Foster-children often feel unheard, unseen, and helpless (Cournos 1999).

Homelessness

Though it does not necessarily mean neglect, the realities and causes of homelessness pose many risks. In addition to loss and grief, there are increased health and safety risks along with reduced access to care (Nabors et al 2004). Children without homes suffer insecurity, and their caregivers may be too overwhelmed to attend to their emotional needs. Depression, posttraumatic stress, illness, disability, poverty, domestic violence, and other life-crises are common among parents of homeless children, all of which can overwhelm parents and reduce their availability. Having no place to call home—in all the forms it takes—can be overwhelming and preoccupying, leaving children anxious and unavailable for learning, wary and worried, angry or withdrawn. Some homeless children can get excessively attached to things and 'overreact' to small losses. Some steal, desperate to have stuff others own. Others may paradoxically seem 'careless' with their things, maybe to have some control over when and how they disappear, maybe because they are not present enough to keep track.

"Her Whole Life in a Plastic Bag"—Tamina: Homelessness and Hunger that Is Not for Food

Tamina attended first grade in a Harlem public school. She was homeless most of that year. Her mother lost the apartment after she lost her job. Sometimes they stayed with relatives but mostly Tamina, her mother, and her sister slept in shelters where they could never stay very long. They carried their belongings in thick black garbage bags, protection from the weather. Tamina used to have a teddy bear, but it got left in a shelter and her mother was 'too tired' to go back for it. Tamina never got it back.

Tamina had very little. Other children had a home, their own bed, place for their stuff, more stuff. So she stole. Mostly small things: erasers, crayons, hairpins. Things she could hide in her pockets and later in her black garbage bag. If confronted, Tamina would furiously demand it "was always hers." I suspected she often believed it and wondered if some items resembled things she once had and owning them was a link to a time when life was less overwhelming. Beyond an overall language delay, Tamina seemed confused about concepts like the difference between possessing and owning: In some shelters cots were 'first-come-first-serve,' and while you had it, it was 'yours' even if it did not remain so for long. You had to 'watch' your stuff or have it disappear. Why could an unattended eraser not be 'hers'?

While children often crave things that are not theirs, Tamina's stealing was possibly about unmet needs. Her mother was "always mad and cussing" and Tamina could not rely on her for support. Children whose 'hungers' are neglected seek other ways: become secretive, dissociate, numb themselves with substances, steal, hoard. These behaviors often further distance them from care and social support, when they in fact communicate confusion, loneliness, anger, loss, and shame.

Caregiver Overwhelm and Inability

The best intentioned caregivers can at times end up inadvertently reinforcing dynamics of isolation and neglect. This is why it is paramount that those working with overwhelmed children understand children's behaviors and the functions they serve and educate and support both children and caregivers. A case in point is that of adoptive parents, who may be unprepared for posttraumatic, dissociative, and attachment reactions in the children. Parents can feel deeply disappointed when the child rejects their love but claims to miss abusive parents or institution life. If difficult behaviors arise, adoptive parents can be alarmed by the child's rage and might end up communicating their fear (and/or regret) to the child in words or actions, reinforcing feelings of rejection and insecurity. Without addressing trauma and dissociation, children's behaviors may be misinterpreted and misdiagnosed, which can lead to failed interventions and possibly the devastation of adoption dissolution. Any subsequent adoption—if it ever happens—will face additional immense challenges. Understanding the dynamics of attachment and trauma (in everyone involved) is why preparation, education, and ongoing support for foster and adoptive parents are crucial, as well as working with the whole family (Bruning 2007, Smith et al 1998).

Family Dynamics and Needs

Distress in a family is never limited to one person. The difficulties of children may be mirroring the family as a whole, and the behaviors of traumatized children can reflect not only past trauma, but also current family issues. Family difficulty may be present and affect others, too, as part of the trauma and/or reaction to it (Deater-Deckard 2005). For example, an ill child may suffer medical trauma, but healthy siblings often endure stress (Janus & Goldberg 1997). There may be less attention, energy, and resources available to them, and parents may be spread too thin to attend sufficiently to their needs. Healthy siblings might minimize their own difficulties and keep overwhelm and worry private, feeling guilty for wanting more when their sibling is not okay. Some struggle with resentment, anger, worry, or grief but if they misbehave or act up they may be chided for "not understanding" or "being selfish." They may end up feeling ashamed for diverting care from the one "who really needs it" and for distressing their parents. They might numb their own feelings and adopt whatever feelings they are expected to have, ignoring their own needs.

"I Try to Be Good"—Elsie: Unseen Sibling

Elsie was eleven and had tongue thrust. Her brother, age seven, was into his second year of cancer treatments. A sitter would drop Elsie off in session, run errands, and pick up the girl on her way back. "I try to be good," Elsie told me in tears during one of our sessions. She had a headache but refused my offer to call her parents for permission to take Tylenol. "I don't want them to worry about me . . ." she said. I responded that her needs mattered too, and fresh tears flowed. "Sometimes I think I'm so good they forget I'm there," she whispered.

Elsie felt guilty if she needed anything; unseen if she needed nothing. She didn't want to "make it worse" for her brother or her parents and so she did not tell them when things were tough at school or when a best friend moved away. She minimized her own discomfort when she felt sick and had a hard time identifying her own emotions. "I know what I'm supposed to say I'm feeling," she told me, "but it feels like I'm lying about it but I don't know what else to say."

Strain and difficulties are frequent among siblings of sick children, as well as in children whose parent is ill, disabled, or in chronic pain. Children can feel guilty for any worsening of the parent's illness, and responsible for regulating the parent's feelings or energy. They may learn to walk on eggshells or withhold their own emotions and needs (Evans & de Souza 2008, Evans et al 2006). Similarly, children of parents who suffer depression and PTSD can find themselves frightened by and for a parent who withdraws or gets triggered into numbness or panic. The children themselves may suffer increased anxiety and depression but work hard to prevent dismay or distress in the parent, becoming hypervigilant of the parent's mood and adapting their needs to accommodate it (Daud et al 2005, Lyons-Ruth & Block 1996, Ostrowski et al 2007).

Familial distress does not need to mean trauma to the child. Many families with illness, crises, or trauma history encourage resilience and growth by maintaining sensitive and effective communication that ensures that everyone is supported and that all have room for their own feelings and needs (Evans & de Souza 2008, Levendosky et al 2003). Nonetheless it is important to keep aware that illness or stress in a family increases a child's risk for secondary stress and unintended neglect, and that overwhelm in all within a family should be assessed.

Child Abuse—Inescapable Realities

Child abuse includes physical abuse, sexual abuse, and emotional abuse. All forms of child abuse occur throughout childhood, with prevalence of physical abuse tending to peak in infancy and early childhood, and then again during the teen years. Sexual abuse risk is highest among little girls ages three to four but occurs both earlier and later in childhood and adolescence, affecting both boys and girls. The prevalence of emotional abuse—the trickiest to define and report—increases steadily with the child's age, in part because of cumulative effects and in part because the risk for emotional abuse grows as children become older (US-DHHS 2013a).

Disability and Abuse

Children are at high risk for abuse if they have chronic medical conditions, congenital and developmental disorders, and intrauterine exposure to drug and alcohol (Crosse et al 1993, Sullivan & Knutson 1998, Sullivan et al 1991, Sullivan et al 2009). Parental mental illness, domestic violence, war, and traumatic loss also increase a child's risk for abuse. In fact, the more risk factors children have, the more vulnerable they are to maltreatment. The increased risk for abuse in these children with special needs may be in part due to parental disappointment, frustration, and difficulty attaching to an imperfect child, as well as the challenges inherent in caring for a special-needs child, which may overwhelm caregivers, who might take it out on the child. Children with communication disorders are more likely to be physically and sexually abused than children without these disorders (Crosse et al 1993, Knutson & Sullivan 1993). Even when parents are not abusive, everyday environments can be overwhelming enough for some children who have an underlying mood disorder, cognitive disorder, or pervasive developmental disorder to suffer posttraumatic and dissociative symptoms (Silberg 1998).

Individuals with disabilities are over four times as likely to be victims of crime as the nondisabled population, with multiple disabilities increasing their risk. For all types of maltreatment, children with disabilities have an up to ten times higher incidence of maltreatment than children without disabilities (Benedict et al 1990, Crosse et al 1993, Goldson 1998, Sullivan & Knutson 2000, Sullivan et al 2009). Disability makes children easy prey for perpetrators and increases maltreatment risk by caregivers (and educators) who lack skills or resources to care for a special-needs child. Raising a disabled child can be exhausting. It can trigger rage, frustration, and overwhelm that can result in damaging behaviors. Among disabled children, those who have difficulty reciprocating affection are at an even higher risk for abuse, as are those with oversensitivities and difficulty regulating emotions. Caregivers can feel that no matter what they do, the child still 'misbehaves' or 'does not respond.' Confusion, helplessness, and frustration can become a self-amplifying feedback loop.

Speech, language, and hearing disorders increase abuse risk and decrease likelihood of disclosure. For example, deaf children are more vulnerable to neglect and emotional, physical, and sexual abuse than hearing children (Sullivan et al 1987). Sexual abuse is especially prevalent, with 50% of deaf girls reporting having been sexually abused compared with 25% of hearing girls, and 54% of deaf boys reporting sexual abuse compared with about 10% in boys with normal hearing (Sullivan et al 1987). Deaf children are less able to fend for themselves and may be less likely or able to 'tell.' Authority figures may not speak sign-language, and marginalization and stigma of hearing loss may cause even deaf children who 'tell' to be misunderstood. Deaf children may have reduced intelligibility and lower language skills, which can complicate disclosure and result in communication failure.

Autism places children at high risk for trauma and abuse (Hershkowitz et al 2007, Sullivan & Knutson 2000). Their risk for overwhelm and confusion is already high due to limited social skills, rigidity, literal thinking, and low threshold for anxiety. They may be unable to put into words what is happening or know how to tell someone about it. Even if they try to disclose, their perception of emotions can be awkward and their narrative can be idiosyncratic, resulting in miscommunications. Because the symptoms of autism can sometimes mimic posttraumatic presentation, people may miss symptoms of posttraumatic stress in autistic children. It can be difficult to discern whether something happened or the autism itself prompted or worsened a behavior.

Sensory integration issues, hypersensitivities, and difficulty regulating are often seen in autism but can affect non-autistic children too (e.g. fetal alcohol syndrome, ADHD, auditory processing disorder). For these children, even normal-range experiences (e.g. a noisy room, strong light or scents) can be overstimulating and may bring on staring, rocking, tantrums, screaming, or self-harm. The behaviors themselves increase risk for abuse, as well as mask posttraumatic responses if adults do not realize that the behaviors are about distress from abuse. Missing such a cue can lead to abuse continuing and dissociation becoming reinforced.

In all children—and especially in disabled children—awareness of the child's history is crucial because of its relation to developmental risks and the host of future problems that may ensue (see Part 3). Trauma is associated with depression and anxiety, dissociation, suicidal and self-destructive behaviors, sexualized behavior, somatization, substance abuse, health issues, eating disorders, impulsivity, aggression, conduct problems, criminal behaviors, cognitive issues, language issues, school problems, attention deficit and hyperactivity, affect-regulation problems, and disturbances in self-concept (Beverly et al 2008, Cole et al 2005, Ford & Courtois 2013, Gaensbauer 2011, Gomez 2012, Heller & Lapierre 2012, Herman 1997, Jamora et al 2009, Kagan 2004, Kendall-Tackett 2002, Levine & Maté 2010, Liotti 2009, Miller 2005, Nadeau & Nolin 2013, Nijenhuis 2004, Putnam 1997, Schore 2001, Siegel 2012, Silberg 1998, 2013, van der Hart et al 2006, van der Kolk 2014, Waters 2005, Wieland 2011). Intervention should not only target behaviors and delays but include understanding of what the behaviors and delays may be communicating about the child's experience and coping.

Domestic Violence

Exposure to domestic violence damages children (Edleson 1999, Sousa et al 2011). Witnessing violence impacts children as much—and sometimes more—than being hit, possibly because of the helplessness that is a hallmark of trauma. Children are helpless to save the caregivers whom they need for survival, let alone when the one harming a caregiver is another someone the child depends on. Caught between a frightening parent and a frightened parent, the child is unable to stop one or save the other.

In addition, domestic violence often renders caregivers unavailable or unable to function due to injury or overwhelm (Levendosky et al 2003, Sousa et al

2011). This can further terrify children who may convince themselves that the violence—and its prevention—is somehow theirs to control. Children often take on blame for what happens: If Mom got hit because dinner wasn't ready, it 'has to be their fault' for asking for Mom's help earlier. In children's minds, if only they were better, quieter, more well behaved, and less needy, the people they rely on would not become terrified or terrifying. Domestic violence is rarely about a real cause, and children may struggle to define one. Maybe they wanted something, or made noise, or wore the wrong color shirt . . .

The very words said during domestic violence can be confusing (e.g. Dad hitting Mom and saying "You happy now? You got me all angry and now look what you made me do!"), leaving the child uncertain of what feelings are or how to understand their own. Shutting down and dissociating are frequent responses to witnessing domestic violence, and children can appear unaffected by a parent's bleeding or painful crying out. They can seem unmoved, unemotional, and numb. They may use aggression themselves, mimicking what they see. Seeing aggression teaches aggression, and reminders of it can activate the same reactions (Gaensbauer 2002, 2011). Traumatized children can react to raised voices as if to violence; they may see a raised arm and cringe; they may raise their own to others when upset or scared. They may hit savagely at the smallest provocation. It may be the only way they learned to respond. They often use actions instead of words or repeat derogatory language. They may have no words to describe what they are doing, how they are feeling, and why.

"She Learn What She Seen"—Lizzie: Seeds of Aggression, Mountains of Fear

Elizabeth (Lizzie), age nine, lived with her mother at her aunt's house along with her four cousins, ages twelve, ten, and five-year-old twins. Before living with the relative, Lizzie and her mom would frequently stay with various friends of her mother's—places the mom fled to when Lizzie's father became violent. Time and again he found them, apologized, and promised to not "get like that again," and they returned home with him; till the next time. Finally when Lizzie was six her mother left for good to a domestic-violence shelter. They moved from shelter to shelter to avoid being found, until Lizzie's father was convicted and put in jail, and the girl and mother could come out of hiding.

By the time I met her, Lizzie had lived at the relatives for two years. These were the safest and most stable years she had ever had, but the past still left its mark. The third grader struggled in school. She had a language/learning delay and attention and impulsivity issues. She had missed much schooling in kindergarten and first grade, but her delays went deeper than catching up. Sweet and friendly most of the time, Lizzie was easily startled. Fidgety and inattentive, her teacher noted "she listened to everything but what relates to class . . . "

Lizzie found it easier to attend in the small speech group. She loved being read to but hated answering questions about what was read, forgot most details, and tried to change the topic to music videos or TV. Fleeting through tasks and skimming through the days, Lizzie was simultaneously disengaged and hypervigilant. Her teeth showed signs of longtime grinding. Never a petite child, Lizzie was taller and heavier than most students her age. She began showing early signs of puberty. She also unveiled a cruel and bullying side: causing a child to smear his/her painting, tripping kids, or pushing them into table corners. Sneaky but outwardly compliant with adults, Lizzie was rarely caught, but when she was, appeared indifferent and shrugged a bland "sorry." She claimed any discipline as "not fair" and that she was "in trouble for nothing." She also seemed surprised when children avoided her after she was cruel to them. In her world, you just said 'sorry' and others had to say it was okay . . .

As Lizzie's aggression escalated, the school threatened expulsion and the mother and aunt showed up for a meeting. The mother sat deflated and silent but the aunt demanded counseling, not expulsion. When the principal claimed that Lizzie's behavior was "simply unacceptable," Lizzie's relative glowered. "Do you know what that child been through?" she challenged. The principal muttered "some domestic violence background" but that he understood things were "fine now." "They sure better," the aunt conceded, undeterred, "but that don't change that she learn what she seen."

Thanks to her aunt's advocacy, Lizzie received counseling at school and her behavior improved some. She progressed academically and in language, but she remained distracted and did best working one-on-one with an adult. The school counselor's only focus was day-to-day behavior management. However, he was empathetic to what Lizzie had endured and was a positive model, if only via providing her an example of a gentle man which countered what she'd seen of male behavior toward females. He and I both wondered whether Lizzie's escalating aggression was related to her preemptively ensuring that no one 'mess with her' (i.e. how her dad hurt her mother), especially as how aggression was what she saw from those larger than others.

Physical Abuse

Physical abuse inflicts terror and pain on the child by the very hands they rely on for love and comfort. Rather than providing safety, caregivers become sources of danger and fear. Even if they are not constantly abusive, caregiver abuse is traumatizing and deeply confusing (Liotti 2004, Lyons-Ruth et al 2006, Silberg 2013). What is a child to do when the person you need frightens you? How can children differentiate care and harm when the same hands dole both? How can a child manage rage when it cannot be safely expressed? What can they make of "love" and "care" when those may (also) mean pain and shame? If small mistakes result in terror, how can a child learn? Who can they turn to? How would they know how?

Children need their caregivers. To preserve connection with caregivers, children will sever their connection to their own experience by dissociating their own feelings, numbing their bodies, trying to anticipate the caregivers' moods, and blaming themselves when abuse happens (Gomez 2012, Silberg 1998, 2013, Wieland 2011). Abused children become hypervigilant to cues for possible danger. Some may act out in ways they know will get them 'punished' because that gives them some sense of control and can reduce the anxiety of awaiting the next explosion. They may not know any other way to connect or get attention. Abuse may be what they believe they deserve.

Many abused children do not talk about what happens. Some do not know how: The child's experience of abuse is rarely explained or put in words. However, even children who possess sufficient language to disclose may believe (or be warned) that telling is forbidden. Children often believe that they do not deserve help and have no reason to trust help will come. They are more likely to trust that worse may follow if they talked.

Not telling does not mean that abused children do not communicate distress. They do: in bruises and injuries, in recoiling, in aggression toward others, in shutting down, in acting out (Pearce & Pezzot-Pearce 1997, Silberg 2013, Waters 2005, Yehuda 2005, 2011)—in what they do not say or talk about; in what they cannot do; in how they talk about themselves, in how they don't. Because fear suppresses exploration and squelches language, we must listen to what they are saying without words (Siegel 2012, van der Kolk 2014). When they do try to tell, it is paramount we hear them—it may be the only time they gather courage to do so. Our reaction may become the yardstick by which they measure whether help will come and whether they are even worth it.

"I Mess Up"—Stephanie: The Justification of Pain

Stephanie was eight. Pretty and popular, she was always surrounded by classmates. Her individualized education plan attributed her marked language delays to English as a second language (Spanish at home), but in reality Stephanie had received English education since preschool. Usually very well behaved, Stephanie could fly into rages with little provocation, then find it difficult to explain what happened, becoming morose and defeated. One time she came to session right after a fight with a classmate. She worried the school would call her mom and told me she didn't want to go home, but when I asked gently what would happen if she got in trouble at home, she just shrugged and said, "Nothing . . ." I told her I was sorry she was struggling and reminded her that if she ever needed to talk to me—about school or home or anything—she could. She gave me a long and suspicious look. Over the following weeks, we spent time in Speech working on verbalizing problem solving, explaining cause-and-effect, and predicting outcomes; all things she and her group-mate struggled with. Stephanie seemed guarded yet curious and I often caught her looking at me when she thought I didn't see.

Then one day she took the chair next to me, leaving the chair across the table for the other student. She seemed on edge and kept shifting in her seat, but when I asked about it, she said that everything was okay. I kept an eye on her, and toward the end of the session noticed the hem of her skirt was lifted, exposing her upper left thigh. There was a large welt on it, angry red and raised. It looked like a burn. Stephanie would not meet my eyes, but she left the skirt up a moment longer before adjusting it. She was trying to show me she was hurt.

I sent the other student back to class. Once alone with Stephanie, I thanked her for showing me her leg. "What happened?" I asked. She stiffened and said, "I mess up." I wondered if she could say more. She hesitantly added she had spilled juice while her mother was cooking and that her mother "got mad." Stephanie fretted whether she was in trouble for showing me, and I reassured her she was not in trouble with me at all, that I was glad she did and that it was very brave of her, and the right thing to do. She looked at me intently, and I asked if there was anything else she wanted to tell me. She shook her head but then raised the edge of her shirt, revealing a tennis-ball size bruise on her lower ribs. It seemed a few days old. "My mommy," she hesitated, demonstrated, "she push me on the door because I clean too slow . ."

It took tremendous courage for Stephanie to show me what was done to her, and more courage to try and explain how and why. Even if no one ever warns them not to tell, children often take it upon themselves to protect their family by keeping the secret that loved ones hurt them. To tell is to risk shame. It makes what one hoped was not real, real. Yet somehow Stephanie managed to show me. Maybe my assurances that she could talk to me had helped. Maybe our recent weeks' language work gave her words to explain. What mattered was that she understood she did the right thing by telling me, by telling someone. I repeated how sorry I was she was hurt, how it was not okay for her to be hurt this way, even if someone was angry. I asked her if she was hurting anyplace else, if there was anything more she wanted to tell or show me, and she shook her head and cried a bit, leaning into me for a hug. She then held my hand and we went to the nurse, where Stephanie got some ice for her welt and let the nurse peek at the bruise on the ribs, not letting go of my hand.

When the nurse asked her how it happened, Stephanie shrugged and looked down: Just because a child disclosed to one person doesn't mean the child will feel safe repeating it to others. The nurse didn't push. She raised an eyebrow at me, and I nodded—we both knew it had to be reported to Child Protection Services—any such mark on a child is reason enough. I walked Stephanie to her class and when I checked on her later she wiggled a shy wave.

CPS made a visit that very day, urged by the dual report and the presence of a young sibling who could also be at risk. Both children were found to have bruises, and a social worker got involved. I don't know what led the mother to use violence against the children, but she enrolled in parenting classes and attended family sessions with the children, who each also got a volunteer 'big brother' and 'big sister.' Stephanie was visibly calmer. She fought less and listened more. She told me things

were "lots better" and that her mom "said sorry" and was "not mean like before"
anymore. I kept reminding Stephanie how much she had helped and can always tell
someone, and she would blush and lean into a hug . . . Stephanie found a way to tell.
Her courage not only saved herself and her sibling but probably their mother, too.

Sexual Abuse and Exploitation

There is little need to explain why sexual abuse—by rape, fondling, or any
exploitation—can be traumatic. When an adult uses a child for sexual gratification, it is not about the child's needs but about the adult. Children can neither
give consent nor understand what it is about. While they have no choice or culpability no matter how the exploitation unfolded, children often blame themselves and feel ashamed, guilty, dirty, broken, and wrong (Gomez 2012, Herman
1997, Lehman 2005, Putnam 1997, Silberg 2013, Wieland 2011). It is obvious
that if there was pain and violence, abuse took place. However, even if there was
no pain; even if the child's body responded; even if the child touched an adult
in curiosity or to receive affection, attention, or a treat; even if the child enjoyed
some of the interest and closeness—sexual exploitation of children remains
abuse.

Sexual abuse is secretive and often contradictory to what a child understands
to be okay. It is rarely narrated or explained (though it might be somehow justified by an abuser), and it leaves no room for the child's experience, feelings,
or needs (Lehman 2005). Being sexually exploited is often confusing and many
children manage that confusion by dissociating from what is happening. They
numb their bodies and feelings, forget, pretend it is happening to someone else,
self-blame, shut down, or act out (Pearce & Pezzot-Pearce 1997, Putnam 1997,
Silberg 2013, Wieland 2011). They have no other choices: They cannot afford to
acknowledge what is taking place, especially when over 90% of children are sexually abused by people they know, and for more than 75% sexual exploitation is
by a parent or close family member (US-DHHS 2013a). What are children to do
when they are used by the people they depend on and need? How can they find
words for what was never worded? How can they disclose and risk more loss and
possibly harm to those they love when they believe it is their fault and that this is
what 'they are good for'? If exploitation and care collided, how does one identify
or trust safety and love?

"Who Knows What that Baby Gone Through"—Marcy: When Trauma Has No Words

Marcy lived with her mother and grandmother, the parents were divorced and origi-
nally shared custody. However, Marcy's father was arrested when she was two when
the mother called police about bruising on the child's genitals after a visitation, and

the police found child pornography on the dad's computer. He reportedly admitted to sharing pictures with others of 'similar interests' and to taking "potentially inappropriate" photos of the child, but denied ever "interfering with her." The police and Marcy's mother were pretty certain that he had, even if forensics could not rule out other causes for the genital findings. The father was convicted on child pornography charges, sent to jail, and ordered to register as a sex offender. The mother was awarded sole custody.

When I saw Marcy, she was four years old and attending preschool. She had language delays and social issues, inattention, inappropriate behavior (compulsive masturbation, aggression), and difficulties with emotional regulation and toileting. She had daytime enuresis and encopresis which after ruling out physical issues were attributed to "issues with control." Marcy's mother agreed the child knew how "to get her way" but worried that the problems related to what she believed had happened to Marcy. "Everyone tells me she was too young to know what he did," she told me, "but I'm not so sure. Who knows what that baby gone through?"

Children may not have cohesive verbal memories of things that happened during infancy and early toddlerhood, but that does not mean their bodies do not remember or that they are not affected by what took place when they were very young (Attias & Goodwin 1999, Brewin 2005, Cozolino 2006, Fogassi & Ferrarri 2007, Gaensbauer 2002, 2011, Heller & Lapierre 2012, Schore 2001, Siegel 2012, van der Kolk 2014). Marcy's behaviors and symptoms spoke of overwhelm and possible reenactment. Many toddlers discover their bodies, and many well-cared-for children masturbate; however, excessive masturbation can be related to trauma, anxiety, and/or sensory issues. Marcy also seemed extraordinarily interested in men and their groins. As toddlers discover that genitalia is different between boys and girls, they can indeed get curious about cataloging who is 'girl' and who is 'boy' by what one does or does not 'have' but are rarely occupied with adult genitalia. Marcy's behavior embarrassed her mother and made male relatives and neighbors uncomfortable, resulting in both implicit and explicit rejection that only added confusion and stress.

While it was quite possible that some of Marcy's issues were rooted in past abuse, there was also the stress of the mother's hyperawareness of her daughter's genitals and behaviors. Marcy probably did not have much verbal memory of what took place in infancy. She certainly did not have sufficient language to verbalize her body's reactions and feelings. Nor was she able to interpret her mother's anxieties when the father's exploitation was discovered, or her mother's conflicting attention, rejection, and shaming since. Marcy was sexually used, and whether she was physically invaded or not, pornography proved the exploitation. Her mother's devastation about it had to be overwhelming to both mother and child. Marcy was expected to stop behaviors that distressed others without understanding why she did these or alternate ways to manage her own activation. Occupied as she was with her body, Marcy's communications and abilities to learn, verbalize, and socialize all suffered.

Verbal Abuse, Emotional Abuse, and Bullying

How we speak to children becomes who they believe they are and can become. Children who are cherished tend to grow up trusting that they are worthy and that people will be there for them. Abusive words produce the opposite, but children have no way to challenge the painful statements: The adults are a child's reality. Emotionally abused children often believe that they are nothing, 'ruin everything,' and cannot do anything right and that it would have been better had they never been born. They learn to not ask for help and may believe they don't deserve it anyway.

Verbal and emotional abuse increases risk for social, relational, psychological, developmental, and health issues (Cole et al 2005, Cozolino 2006, Denham 1998, Freyd & Birrell 2013, Heineman 1998, Jamora et al 2009, Lyons-Ruth & Block 1996, Netherton et al 1999, Pearce & Pezzot-Pearce 1997, Perry & Szalavitz 2006, Siegel 2012, Silberg 2013, van der Kolk 2014). Emotionally abused children often replay old patterns. People who were themselves raised in an abusive home may reenact it on others, resulting in verbal and emotional abuse repeating through generations (Haapasalo & Aaltonen 1999). Learned patterns of abuse can also be mirrored in children's interactions as victims and perpetrators of bullying (Eliot & Cornell 2009, Espelage et al 2000). In some ways all emotional abuse is bullying, and bullying is abuse. Awareness of its seriousness has increased recently following tragedies of children who took their own lives—or the lives of others—after being bullied and/or cyberbullied (Hinduja & Patchin 2010).

Even if they do not resort to taking lives, bullied children often use numbing, self-harm, addiction, and dissociation to manage the devastation of being emotionally abused. Being a bully is also associated with increased risk for mental illness, social adjustment, and criminality. One way bullying is traumatizing may be that bullying impact can be invisible and difficult to define, with bullying still being trivialized, minimized, denied, deflected, and dismissed. This further invalidates a child's feelings and increases confusion and isolation. With no place to go with their fear, rage, and confusion, children who are bullied may dissociate or act out these feelings with others or on themselves, perpetuating pain.

As with other emotional abuse cycles, those involved with bullying—bullies as well as bullied—often have maltreatment histories, which makes addressing bullying doubly important. In a longitudinal study of adults who had been part of a research cohort since they were children in the 1950s, Takizawa et al (2014) found that childhood bullying—especially prolonged—was associated with depression, social difficulties, anxiety, cognitive difficulties, and suicidality. These difficulties persisted into later life (age 45–50) and were on a par with those of children who had grown up in foster-care and experienced multiple adverse childhood events. Bullying was also associated with low educational outcomes and subsequent economic disparity. Those who were bullied as children tended to have low parental involvement, higher incidence of foster placements, and additional childhood adversities.

Maltreatment and bullying form a vicious cycle: Being maltreated places children at a high risk for bullying when these are the children who have fewer resources for coping with the bullying when it takes place. The stresses of being maltreated—and/or bullied—keep children from learning, attending, and succeeding and place them at a risk for continued cycles of stress and adversity. Bullying should serve as a red flag for a child in overwhelm.

"It Was Another Boy"—Charlie and Bill: Bullying and Abuse

By the time Charlie's parents found out he was being bullied, it had been going on for some time. A teacher caught the bully (and his cronies) twisting nine-year-old Charlie's arm and hanging him on a doorknob by the back of his underwear. The torment had apparently been daily. Charlie's parents were shocked: He never complained and did not appear to hate school (though he often suffered stomachaches and left school early).

When asked about it, Charlie denied the bullying happened. "Oh, it didn't happen to me," he stated calmly. "It was another boy." His parents were flabbergasted— the teacher had lifted him off the doorknob, yet Charlie appeared to believe that none of it had happened to him. Small for his age, Charlie had been adopted at birth, needed many therapies to catch up, and was in Speech with me for language and processing issues. He spaced out a lot in class and I wondered if he might have dissociated during bullying episodes.

Rather than calling for punishment of the bullies, Charlie's parents urged the school to teach empathy, increase understanding to what bullying is about, and assess the history of the bullies to ensure that they were not hurting. With Charlie's permission, his parents arranged a schoolwide presentation where they shared how he was "chosen" (i.e. adopted), how hard he worked to grow, and his robot-building awards. The students were impressed, but Charlie's parents did not stop there. They engaged the students in speaking about how bullying makes children feel (weak, unimportant, sad, lonely) and how bullies might feel (powerful, strong, important, in control), and asked why students thought a child might need to feel that way by being mean to another. The children's responses were illuminating: "someone was mean to them" or "he don't feel good about himself," etc.

After the assembly, a student told a teacher that Bill, Charlie's main bully, was "being mean to at home," that Bill's father kept saying he was "a good-for-nothing kid," and put him down for not "being a man in wrestling" against the adult. So, it was no big surprise that Bill learned to exert physical power over a smaller person to feel powerful. He may have felt jealous of Charlie, who was so clearly adored, getting what Bill couldn't get . . .

The two boys never became friends but the bullying did stop. It was no longer 'cool' to bully when children got more social power from being 'friend protectors' than bullies. Charlie's parents avoided vilifying the bully and used empathy to help students see cruelty as a cry for help. I don't know if the torment by Bill's parent was proven or resolved, but hopefully his pain was at least somewhat ameliorated by the school's ego-building support.

Children like Bill who struggle to develop empathy need help. Empathy is part of healthy connection. Its lack can communicate the 'rules' a child had internalized about the world and feelings. Improving empathy can help reduce bullying and address its causes. This also includes informing faculty (and parents) about factors that inadvertently foster bullying atmospheres: playing favorites, upholding perfection, teaching that "win and you're a Winner, lose and you are a Loser," creating hierarchies, etc. A 'zero tolerance' to bullying should not mean shaming the bullies. Rather it should address bullying as requiring action and as an opportunity to identify vulnerable children who may be carrying hurts that need attending to and that may be diverting much of their energy away from growth and learning.

6 The Neuroscience of Trauma, Emotional Regulation, and the Developing Self

Interest in children's development is not new. However, practical and ethical limitations kept most investigations of neurological, anatomical, and functional brain development to animal models or theoretical speculations. It is only recently that advances in non-invasive imaging have opened opportunities for studying children's brain development and the impact of environmental and interpersonal factors. More time may be needed before imaging studies can offer longitudinal maturational data, but research already allows insight into neurological, neuro-physiological, cognitive, regulatory, chemical, and anatomical development in children. Excellent resources for in-depth study of neuroscience and neurodevelopment are available (Cozolino 2006, 2014, Gaensbauer 2002, 2011, Levine & Maté 2010, Scaer 2014, Schore 2012, Siegel 2012, van der Kolk 2014, to name a few), and the summary of this chapter is meant as but a glancing overview of a complex and specialized topic.

Brain Growth, Hemispheric Integration, and Development

The early years are characterized by magnificent growth that takes place concurrently in multiple and highly interrelated systems. Children's experiences and their reactions to them both form and link to regulatory systems (e.g. the hypothalamic–pituitary–adrenal axis) and build neurological 'highways' for recognition, response, and regulation of body states, arousal, and affect (Cozolino 2006, Gaensbauer 2002, 2011, Schore 2012, Siegel 2012, van der Kolk 2014). It is nothing short of magical that children simultaneously develop motor control, sensory processing, affective expression and perception, comprehension and expression, social cognition, empathy, world concepts, self-perception, and complex relational abilities. Throughout development, early experiences, reactions, communication, language, affect, and regulation are deeply interconnected.

Children's brains show phenomenal growth and maturation in the first few years of life, with all areas of the brain growing, interacting, sheathing, and connecting (Cozolino 2006, Knickmeyer et al 2008, Choe et al 2013, van der Kolk

2014). The brain is an integrated system of structures, including the right and left hemispheres, the corpus callosum that connects them, the left and right cerebellum, the brainstem, limbic system, and more. Though most sensory and motor information is processed and controlled contralaterally (e.g. the left hemisphere controls movement of the body's right side, and vice versa), there is much crossover and integration between structures on both sides of the brain (Choe et al 2013, Knickmeyer et al 2008, van der Kolk 2014).

While growth takes place throughout the brain, there is some asymmetry in growth during the first years of life, with certain structures being larger on the left (e.g. cerebrum, globus, pallidus, lateral ventricle, cerebellar hemisphere), others being larger on the right (caudate, hippocampus, ventral diencephalon); and some that switch symmetry from left to right (putamen) (Choe et al 2013). Specialization and dominance also become more pronounced, with areas on one side becoming particularly 'good' at managing certain tasks or stimuli (e.g. some locations in the left hemisphere correlate with language processing and producing speech, while corresponding areas in the right hemisphere correlate with expressive and receptive abilities for face recognition, emotion, pace, pitch, symbolic meaning, and nonverbal aspects of communication) (Balsamo et al 2008, Cozolino 2006, Schore 2012). That said, hemispheric dominance does not imply exclusivity, absoluteness, or separateness: Information crosses over continuously between hemispheres, and processing requires ongoing integration between the hemispheres and other structures. The formation of pathways and coordination between the two sides of the brain is especially crucial in children, whose brains and hemispheric specializations are still developing (Balsamo et al 2008, Knickmeyer et al 2008, Teicher et al 2004, van der Kolk 2014).

Different areas of the brain show accelerated growth and maturation at different ages, but all areas grow and participate in integration and processing of information throughout development. Normally developing babies move both sides of their bodies and perceive the world through both eyes/ears/hands/feet/nostrils and both sides of their tongue and mouth. As information flows into the nervous system from throughout the baby's body, sensory fibers travel through the brainstem, medulla, cerebellum, and cortex. They are processed by many areas of the brain simultaneously (or with infinitesimal time lag for localization or processing, as in the development of right ear advantage for language processing) (Bryden et al 1983).

Brain Development and Maltreatment

An infant's world revolves around sensation and internal states, feedback, interaction, and connection. Input and response become the basis for meaning and regulation and make brain development intrinsically related to attachment and communication. It also explains why trauma and maltreatment affect it so significantly (Cozolino 2006, Gaensbauer 2002, Levine & Maté 2010, Scaer 2014, Schore 2012, Siegel 2012, van der Kolk 2014).

When a mother smiles, talks to, and gently touches the baby during baby-care, multiple areas of the brain are bilaterally activated. The visual pathways and the visual cortexes activate and make connections to facial recognition areas, memory areas, mirror-neurons, and motor areas. The auditory pathways and the auditory cortexes activate to process hearing, attend to and identify inflection, recognize voice, tone, speech sounds, and later on words and meaning. Memory areas interconnect with facial recognition, visual areas, and motor areas to form an integrated sense of what makes the sound and how. Sensory areas on both sides activate to process and respond to the tactile stimulation from the mother's touch, the fabric as it slides on or off the infant's body, the temperature of the air, the coolness of the wet-cloth, the dryness of the clean diaper, the softness of the mother's stroke, etc. Motor areas activate to move arms, eyes, legs, and lips. All these happen simultaneously to create an interconnected experience: the sensa-tions, the sounds, the smells, the visuals, and the associations between the moth-er's facial movements, smile, and tone and the baby's own movements, smile, and voice. Multitudes of activated neurons 'fire together' and 'wire together' in the experience of being in the vicinity of the mother and being cared for by her. Neurotransmitters of well-being and connection 'bathe' the brain. As such care repeats in its myriad variations, these connections are reinforced and weave the experience of care with regulation, comfort, safety, and pleasure.

Unfortunately, when less favorable experiences happen, they are also multisen-sory and multi-activating, forming their own associations and connections. If a caregiver is angry, hurtful, ignoring, or abusive, these experiences become 'wired into' the baby's brain along with the chemical, hormonal, physiological, and affec-tive connections the experience formed. Here, too, repetitions will reinforce con-nections, associations, and responses: of alarm, tension, overwhelm, fear, pain (Cozolino 2006, Gaensbauer 2011, Scaer 2014, Schore 2012, van der Kolk 2014).

Infants may not yet have the language to comprehend or express a traumatic experience, but their brains still get activated by it. Voice, tone, background noises, and words activate auditory and language areas, get encoded in somatic memory, and become connected with the visual information of a caregiver's glower or frown (Gaensbauer 2011). Sensory information from the infant's body, along with the flooding of affect, discomfort, pain, and overwhelm, 'bathe' the baby's brain in stress hormones. As activation from the stimuli becomes connected with such flooding, networks of reactions are formed and reinforced (Scaer 2014, van der Kolk 2014).

The nervous system is part of the much bigger system of the organism. Immune responses, hormonal responses, gut responses, and visceral and auto-nomic and vaso-vagal responses all take place in reaction to activation (Felitti et al 1998, Scaer 2014, van der Kolk 2014). Throughout life, for good or bad, we are in constant interrelation with our internal environment, external environment, and other persons. Depending on the quality of these interactions and a child's abilities (and help) with regulating the experience of these interactions, the brain responds, grows, learns, and changes.

Anatomical—the Effects of Stress on Brain Growth

Though the brain reaches maturation in adulthood, it is a dynamic organ that continues to form and prune connections through the lifespan. During embryonic development, infancy, childhood, adolescence, and early adulthood, different areas of the brain show periods of relatively rapid maturation (Choe et al 2013, Knickmeyer et al 2008). The accelerated growth of a particular area (or several overlapping areas) is often associated with the specific tasks that are the hallmark of a particular time period (Balsamo et al 2008).

Brain structures undergoing rapid growth are vulnerable to disruptions and delays, and traumas at different ages have an increased impact on the brain structures that grow rapidly during that time (Teicher et al 2004, van der Kolk 2014). The neuro-developmental impact of trauma can vary depending on the child's age at the time of the trauma.

The brainstem, responsible for physiological regulation, undergoes rapid maturation immediately after birth (birth to three months), and trauma at this age can affect physiological regulation. The limbic system shows an accelerated rate of maturation between two and six months of age, and the cortico-limbic integration speeds up from around the third month of life through to the eighteenth. The right hemisphere shows relative accelerated growth at about the same time (6–18 months), while the left hemisphere's accelerated growth begins a few months later and continues through the second year (12–24 months). The hippocampus shows rapid growth throughout the first two years of life (0–24 months) and is followed by accelerated growth of intercortical integration via the corpus callosum (24–48 months). The prefrontal cortical development accelerates from the second half of the second year through preschool (18–48 months) (Choe et al 2013, Gaensbauer 2011, Knickmeyer et al 2008, Schore 2012, van der Kolk 2014). This multistructure growth makes infancy and early childhood a crucial time for regulatory, affective, and relational development and explains why trauma in early childhood adversely affects development, and why ongoing trauma affects so many aspects of it.

Accelerated growth in some areas does not preclude growth and maturation of other structures in other areas, and even after accelerated growth slows, maturation continues. All brain structures develop throughout infancy and childhood and can be affected by childhood experiences. What varies is the relative pace (or 'focus') of maturation during different times for different sections of the brain. Brain areas do not represent distinct organs but are parts of an interrelated, interconnected system, where maturation of one area also means increased connections with (and therefore activation of) other areas. Chronic trauma (e.g. neglect, abuse) reinforces posttraumatic reactions and trauma-related feedback loops throughout the brain and prevents other connections from taking place (Gaensbauer 2011, Scaer 2014, Siegel 2012, van der Kolk 2014).

Brains require stimulation and opportunities for experience and learning in order to grow. Children who suffered chronic neglect have smaller brains (less gray matter, less 'folds' in the cortex) than non-neglected peers (van der Kolk 2014). Malnutrition plays a role in retarding growth in some neglected children, but smaller brains were seen in children who were sufficiently fed yet received inadequate interaction. Smaller brain size correlates with reduced abilities in language, cognition, memory, and executive function (Albers et al 2005, Cozolino 2006, Miller 2005).

Even when the overall size of the brain is not diminished, chronic stress may affect brain structures such as the corpus callosum and hippocampus (Teicher et al 2004, Bremmer et al 1997). Studies found smaller left hippocampal volume in patients with posttraumatic stress disorder (PTSD), as well as in persons with schizophrenia, in their nonschizophrenic family members, and in people suffering from depression and anxiety—all groups who experience high stress. Fortunately, there is indication that plasticity can help brain structures recover with intervention that reduces PTSD symptoms and lowers stress (van der Kolk 2014).

Chemical and Metabolic—Formed and Bathed in Stress

Our brain reacts to and controls chemical, metabolic, and physiological changes throughout the body. Any time it responds to stimuli—both pleasant and unpleasant—the brain secretes hormones, endorphins, and neurotransmitters which affect our overall chemistry and physical reactions, as well as our immune system, autonomic system, and metabolism. When stress hormones are released in response to overwhelm, a cascade of stress-related responses unfurls, affecting that child chemically, metabolically, emotionally, cognitively, psychologically, and physiologically. If trauma recurs (and/or trauma reminders reactivate), stress responses accumulate and become reinforced, amplified, and sensitized. The resulting neuro-developmental patterns affect the child's coping and future physiological response. Stress hormones may remain chronically high or may become depleted, leaving the child unable to respond effectively to stress and increasing the risk to both development and health (Cozolino 2006, Felitti et al 1998, Levine & Maté 2010, Siegel 2012, van der Kolk 2014).

Danese et al (2009) conducted a longitudinal study and found that by their early 30s, people who were exposed to adverse childhood experiences were at an elevated risk for depression, high inflammation levels (as measured by high-sensitivity C-reactive protein level >3 mg/L), and clusters of metabolic risk markers (overweight, high blood pressure, high total cholesterol, high glycated hemoglobin, and low maximum oxygen consumption levels). Socioeconomic disadvantage, maltreatment, or social isolation in childhood elevated the disease risks in the adults. Moreover, the effects of adverse childhood experiences were cumulative and independent of the influence of other risk factors. The researchers concluded that adverse psychosocial experiences in childhood have enduring emotional, immune, and metabolic abnormalities that elevate risk for age-related disease. While trauma prevention in children is important either way, the risk (and costs) of disease only reinforce the need to minimize children's exposure to it.

All types of trauma can increase chronic stress and its health impact. Takizawa et al (2014) found that bullying victimization in childhood was associated with cognitive difficulties, anxiety, depression, and poor health outcomes. The authors hypothesized that the problems may be related to findings of blunted cortisol response and higher serotonin transporter gene methylation levels in victims of childhood bullying. Chronic stress may change brain regulation, and/or children with innately weaker regulatory abilities may be more vulnerable to and more affected by stress. Either way, the connections among stress, neurochemistry, psychology, physiology, and regulation are complex and interconnected with genetics and metabolic and relational factors. Research looks at different aspects of trauma, but overwhelm affects the whole child.

Bowlby observed the 'failure to thrive' among institutionalized babies who received physical care but not enough interpersonal care. Both behaviorally and physiologically, the children no longer responded as normal children were expected to. Their bodies shut down. Some died (Bowlby 1997). In his book *Children Who Don't Want to Live*, Orbach (1988) describes depression and even suicidal ideation in very young children. Some children show physical failure to thrive, others may withdraw from curiosity, activity, and communication. Their joy or excitement can seem blunted—their very spark dimmed.

Regulatory—Ineffective 'Volume Control'

Environmental input is usually experienced across several sensory domains simultaneously. Sensitive caregivers ensure that children are not exposed to more than they can tolerate and help children regulate, interpret, and habituate to stimulation (Cozolino 2006, Siegel 2012, Stams et al 2002). Caregiver support is essential, because both understimulation and overstimulation (of any sensory modality) can become overwhelming.

Kinesthetic

To develop healthily, babies require tactile stimulation via affectionate handling, proximity, and holding. Studies on animals and children (e.g. Bowlby's 'failure to thrive' studies), as well as recent orphanage evidence, have repeatedly shown how fundamental touching and holding are to babies' growth (Cozolino 2006, 2014, Miller 2005, Newberry & Swanson 2008, van der Kolk 2014). Babies also need to experience movement in space to stimulate the equilibrium system and the integration of visual and kinesthetic information it involves. The development of infants who spend too long in cribs and too little time in arms and in movement can be hampered (Albers et al 2005, Miller 2005).

Too little stimulation can lead to shut down, as can too much tactile and kinetic stimulation: When babies are handled roughly, shaken, hit, slammed, shoved, burned, scalded, left too cold or too hot, they cannot get away, change the situation, or stop what is happening. All they can do is shut down and numb out, tamping down development and exploration as well (Silberg 2013).

Auditory

Babies must hear language to develop oral language. Language learning can still take place for babies born to deaf parents who use rich sign language with them from birth. However, the children will not learn to speak without hearing language spoken. For the auditory cortex to develop, babies should be exposed to speech and learn to discriminate among sounds, identify them, and give them meaning (Baron 1992, Berman 2004, Gleason & Ratner 2009). When caregivers talk to infants, their tone of voice, intonation, and volume all combine with the caregivers' touch and facial expression and the baby's internal state (e.g. hungry, wet, tired, content) (de Boysson-Bardies 1999, Halla 1999, Nazzi et al 1998, Nelson 1987). This input helps the auditory pathways become part of sensory processing and regulation paths that are integral to learning. Interpretation of sound into meaning is learned: Babies acquire it through being talked to and interacted with in context (Cozolino 2006, 2014, Ninio & Snow 1996). If they do not have the opportunity to do so they may not learn to associate hearing with listening or attending. They may not learn to differentiate background sounds from what needs to be focused on. They may not know how to respond to sounds.

Responding to sounds also includes identifying which sounds require arousal for action or reaction and which allow return to calm. A sudden sound is often startling, but if our brain identifies it as something benign (e.g. a muffler of a passing car), our autonomic system receives the message from our brain that the stimuli does not warrant an alarm, and our bodies calm. If the sound is indeed deemed worthy of alarm, our adrenaline will remain high as we spring into action to either move away (e.g. a honk of a too-close car) or toward the sound (e.g. someone's hard fall). Even then, our arousal can be tempered by our understanding of what is taking place and what needs to be done (van der Kolk 2014). Babies who are not spoken to may become underresponsive (treat all sounds as insignificant) or overresponsive (treat all sounds as potential danger).

Being deprived of language is harmful—so is being yelled at and being exposed to overwhelming sounds that may involve fear and pain to children (e.g. physical abuse or neglect) or to those they depend on (e.g. domestic violence). For these children, attending to sounds may be terrifying. They might dissociate from hearing or become hypervigilant and overreact to neutral sounds as if to danger. They do not respond to auditory stimuli in ways that promote processing, integration, and understanding and may not know to utilize auditory information for attending, listening, and learning (Fox et al 1988, Gaensbauer 2011, Holt et al 2008, Levendosky et al 2003, Levine & Kline 2007, Pearce & Pezzot-Pearce 1997, Silberg 1998, Yehuda 2005).

Taste

Taste preferences can vary among children and are often influenced by culture and exposure. However, taste buds in infants and children are generally more sensitive than in adults, and they are more likely to find strong flavors aversive (Piazza & Carroll-Hernandez 2004). By putting things in their mouths and experimenting with food and nonfood flavors, children desensitize their mouths and increase their repertoire of acceptable flavors and textures. Infants and children who experience too little variety (e.g. institutionalized children who are fed bland uniform food) can have feeding issues, difficulty tolerating new food, increased sensitivity in the mouth, and oral-motor and feeding issues (Albers et al 2005, Miller 2005). Tastes can feel scary to them, even causing gag. On the other end of the continuum are children who were fed food that was too hot, too spicy, spoiled, or foul—as well as the children who were forced to have things in their mouths they did not want (and/or that did not belong there). Tasting can feel overwhelming, and yet they must eat to survive, so children dissociate: They do not taste the food and do not know how to discern what they like and what they don't, what is edible and what is not. The dissociation may extend to other sensations in their mouths, affecting oral-motor and speech development.

Visual

Visual information is crucial for learning spatial relationships and proximity, discovering meaning (e.g. connecting sound to object), attaching (recognizing caregivers' faces), relating (identifying and responding to emotions in facial expressions), and more (Cozolino 2006, 2014, Nelson 1987, Ninio & Snow 1996, Schore 2012). Babies need to experience the world around them in order to be able to assess distance, shape, heft, and structure. By seeing things from many different angles, they learn to infer a whole from a part (e.g. recognize a chair even though most of it is hidden by a table). Visual information allows babies to make connections between what they see, hear, and feel; what they can expect to taste, reach for, refuse, smile at, or push away.

When a baby has too little visual stimulation (e.g. too long in a crib, a dim room, little interaction), the development of the visual cortex and its connections to other areas of the brain can suffer. Children may not know to respond to smiles or how to make eye contact; they may not reach for items or a caregiver's hand (Albers et al 2005, Miller 2005). Overwhelming visual stimulation can also stall development and curtail exploration and attending. Glaring, angry faces are frightening to children. They can become hypervigilant to small changes in facial expression, not knowing which could herald harm (Pollak et al 2000). They might have difficulty knowing what to attend to (i.e. figure/ground) and be anxious about missing something crucial to safety. They may overrespond and obsess over minor details, or shut down and underrespond. Babies might not know how to respond to expressions that are neutral or loving. If eye contact was scary, babies may not make eye contact and instead look away or around people's faces (Gray 2002). They may fixate on something else (e.g. their fingertips, a thread in their shirt) or stare into space (Beverly et al 2008, Miller 2005).

Olfactory

The sense of smell is arguably the most 'evocative' of human senses. Olfactory stimuli connect to and activate our limbic and autonomic systems, which can result in visceral responses and memory activation (Gaensbauer 2011, Wieland 2011). Evolutionarily, scent held life-and-death information (e.g. was there a predator upwind?), and survival required that smell connect directly to past and future experiences. Humans rarely need to identify predators by scent these days but olfactory information remains highly meaningful. Early memories may be smell related and often evoke emotional responses. "The smell of home" can bring up cozy, warm memories or trigger paralyzing terror, depending on the association of that smell. The smell of pinewood may bring up feelings of despair in someone who was abandoned as a baby in an empty pine crate (Renee Potgeiter, personal communication).

Babies rely on adults to put smells in context and alleviate offensive odors. Maltreated babies who were left in their own refuse, fed spoiled milk, or otherwise neglected can find even everyday smells overwhelming. They overreact to small changes in smells and odors and find it difficult to habituate to ongoing smells. They may shut down and appear inured to even noxious odors. Abused children may find all manner of smells frightening: beer breath or perfume like that of the perpetrator, the soap in the bath where they were molested, musty odors like those in the basement they were sent to for punishment, the metallic smell of blood after Dad punched Mom ... Because smell is so visceral, some traumatized children numb themselves to it. Others become hypervigilant, avoid whole categories of smells, or are hypersensitive to even faint scents.

Hypersensitivity and Sensory Integration Issues

Sensory information needs to be integrated with other information to be processed and regulated. Hypersensitivities and difficulties with regulating and integrating information can complicate (or even cause) trauma. A child may have too sensitive a threshold (i.e. the lowest level where stimuli are just detectable) or too low a tolerance (i.e. the highest 'volume' of a stimuli one can tolerate) and find stimulation that barely bothers others intolerable. Other children may have normal sensory thresholds and tolerance but have a hard time habituating to ongoing stimuli (e.g. keep feeling the fabric of clothes, be unable to 'tune out' background noise), attenuating stimuli, differentiating stimuli, or identifying stimuli. They can get overwhelmed because sensations are unremitting and undifferentiated, and they are constantly flooded by mundane sensory data most of us ignore (Barth et al 2000, Degangi & Kendall 2008, Heymann 2010, Miller 2005, Smith & Gouze 2004).

Sensitivity level is partially a matter of biology. However, it can also be affected by limited opportunity for regulation (e.g. abuse, neglect) and/or stimuli that exceed the child's tolerance (e.g. medical trauma). Traumatized children often present with low tolerance and difficulty integrating some sensory information. In some well-cared-for children, oversensitivity and sensory regulation issues can be overwhelming even in the absence of trauma (i.e. children with autism or auditory processing disorder). For a hypersensitive child, even a less-than-responsive caregiver can make life difficult to manage—let alone in cases of maltreatment, where the child's sensory overload is not acknowledged or respected and feelings of helplessness and isolation pile on top of the already flooding experience. The unprocessed sensations may lead to hypersensitization, especially if sensory stimulation came along with intense or repeated pain.

Pain Sensitization

Pain is an information system all its own. It connects to sensory data, visceral data, physiology, perceptions, interpretations, and emotions (Kuttner 2010). Undertreated pain can lead to oversensitization of pain pathways and increase pain reaction later on (hyperalgesia). The immature neurobiology of premature babies, infants, and children makes them vulnerable to developing oversensitization to pain (and other sensory information), as they are less able to modulate and regulate it and are more easily overwhelmed by it (for more information about premature babies and pain in children, see Chapter 4).

Early experiences form the baseline for autonomic and regulatory response to stimuli. Infants whose early experiences have been soothing and calming internalize (neurologically and physiologically) an ability to downregulate from an unsettled place. Their bodies 'know' how to become soothed. Those who experienced pain and overwhelm can take longer to soothe and may find it harder to manage future pain (Anand & Hickey 1987, Browne 2003, Doesburg et al 2013, Simons et al 2003, Varni et al 1996, William et al 2004, WHO 2013). If children risk pain sensitization when in caring medical settings, how much more so when pain comes from neglect and abuse and is almost by definition unacknowledged and undertreated? Traumatized persons often suffer pain, exhibit somatic symptoms, and may use dissociation to cope (Felitti et al 1998, Kendall-Tackett 2002, Nijenhuis 2004, Scaer 2014, Silberg 2013).

Paradoxical Regulation: Self-harm

Self-mutilation and self-harm represent attempts at regulating affect and overwhelm (Silberg 2013, van der Kolk 2014). Though associated with teens, self-harm is not limited to adolescents. Even toddlers can—and do—deliberately self-harm. Some children self-harm to feel alive—they are so numb that they feel compelled to hurt themselves just to feel something or see that they still bleed and therefore are real. Others self-harm for the detachment and numbness that can accompany self-harming behaviors, or for the endorphins that may be released in the process and may bring them some relief. Self-harm is clearly a drastic means of regulation, but desperate children use desperate measures to manage what they cannot bear.

"So I Can Go to the Stars"—Travis

Travis, age eight, pinched himself to bruises by twisting the flesh on the sides of his torso. If 'caught self-mutilating' he was removed to the principal's office and his foster-mother was called to take him home. After he missed a session because he was sent home, I asked him if the pinching helped. He hesitated. I could not blame him: Talking about his self-harm had led to him being suspected of "early psychosis," and the medication that followed made him feel "even more like pinching." Travis' trauma history was well known, but the self-harm began after the boy was in a stable home and so was not seen as trauma related. I thought it quite possible that it was. Travis was removed to foster-care at age three following prolonged neglect by his addicted parents and was abused in his first foster-home. His second foster-home was excellent, but it did not erase his history or its impact.

"It makes the noises in my head more quiet so I can go in the stars," he finally said.

"I can understand how sometimes things like that can help," I replied. He stared at me, then added quietly, "When I get sad my heart gets tight and I can't breathe so I pinch and I go into the stars."

Relational Impact of Sensory Deprivation or Overwhelm

Reaction to sensory information depends on temperament and biology as well as one's experience of care and relational interactions (Cozolino 2006, 2014, Schore 2012, Siegel 2012). While babies differ in what stimulation they find unpleasant, well-cared-for infants learn that distress is temporary and that caregivers can be counted on to alleviate it. This allows them to tolerate discomfort with less alarm and return quickly to baseline (Silberg 2013, van der Kolk 2014). Even in high-distress situations (e.g. injury, illness), children whose parents are calm and calming tend to manage pain and stress better than children whose caregivers are anxious about the child's distress (Browne 2003, Gil et al 1991, Ostrowski et al 2007, Speechley & Noh 1992, Winston et al 2002). The caregivers' ability to meet the child's needs is integral to regulation. It is why maltreated infants, who may have learned that discomfort persists and that others do not help or make it worse, can find even small discomforts alarming. Feeling alarmed worsens the experience of distress and makes it more likely to overwhelm. For a child with many unmet needs, even small lapses in good care or perceived ill-treatment can trigger dissociation as a response to distress (De Bellis 2005, Levine & Kline 2007, Milot et al 2010, Nadeau et al 2013, Shields & Cicchetti 1998, Silberg 2013, Wieland 2011).

Automatic—Where Stress and Language Shall Not Meet

Repeated experiences of alarm, distress, and overwhelm increase the risk for lasting effects on brain development, behavior, and physiology. Age at trauma, frequency, severity, and types of trauma all interact with temperament to compound a child's likelihood for posttraumatic and dissociative activation (Silberg 2013). The areas of the brain that are responsible for language and assimilation of new information are suppressed by increased activity in the areas of the brain that are reactive to stress (van der Kolk 2014). Stress responses lead to deactivation of language centers, impacting processing, memory, comprehension, formulation, and expression. Even adults find it difficult to process trauma until the stress is reduced and the experience can be put in words (Herman 1997)—let alone children, whose language skills are still developing and whose access to the modulating benefit of processing is still limited. For chronically overwhelmed children, this may lead to a vicious cycle of activation, language suppression, confusion, and overwhelm.

Repeated stress activation can lead to hypervigilance, easy startle, irritability, fidgeting, and sleep disturbances—all common in traumatized children. Because of difficulties with regulation, children may seem to 'overreact' or 'underreact' and are often reported to be erratic, intense, disorganized, forgetful, inattentive, detached, apathetic, and unmotivated (Pearce & Pezzot-Pearce 1997, Putnam 1997, Silberg 1998, 2013, Terr 1990, Waters 2005, Yehuda 2004, 2005). These symptoms are often misunderstood and children end up being judged as impulsive, aggressive, willful, and manipulative (Silberg 1998, 2013, Wieland 2011). When they get disciplined for reactions their bodies developed to survive, children understandably feel helpless and alone, which adds to their stress and need for dissociation.

Chronic stress affects multiple bodily systems and disrupts homeostasis (Felitti et al 1998, Kendall-Tackett 2002, Takizawa et al 2014). Our bodies are not meant to remain in a state of high activation: Vigilance and stress are biologically intended as short-term reactions to imminent threat that are widely spaced by periods of calm (van der Kolk 2014). Digestion, immune response, growth, repair, processing and learning all require calm states and are compromised by stress. In children, whose main tasks include learning, exploring, experimenting, and attending, disruption by chronic stress is especially detrimental. Beyond the issues with inattention, memory, processing, and behavior, children often suffer somatic complaints. These may be directly related to the trauma (i.e. pain from injury and trauma reminders activating somatic memory) or represent generalized response to chronic stress (e.g. stomach and digestion issues, headaches, fatigue) (Silberg 2013, Wieland 2011). Without the benefit of processing the traumatic experiences, making meaning and putting them into words, stress becomes locked in the body, reinforcing more distress (Cozolino 2014, Levine & Maté 2010, Scaer 2014, van der Kolk 2014).

We all live in bodies that have physiological reactions to environmental stimuli, internal stimuli, and our interpretations of either. Physiology affects psychology and psychology affects physiology. When we feel happy, our lips relax, our pupils dilate, our heart rate may quicken in pleasure, our energy increases, our digestive system bubbles, and our immune response gets a boost. When we get angry, pulse may rise, skin might flush, and lips can tighten. We can get indigestion or lose our appetite.

Prolonged stress leaves a mark. It shapes children's mind and body, their reaction to everyday stimuli, and sensitivity to additional stress. Children's perception of themselves and the world evolves through the interaction of physiological, biological, and temperamental states, along with the relational experiences children have with caregivers. Trauma—and dissociation—disrupt this process and interferes with the child's ability to organize, make sense of, remember, retrieve, and narrate experiences. In Part 3, the ways trauma can impact language, attention and learning, vocabulary and semantics, and pragmatics and socialization will be detailed along with their clinical implications.

Part 3

The Language of Trauma

7 How Trauma Affects Language and Why It Matters So Much More in Children

Ten-month-old Millie is sitting in her stroller as her mother talks with a neighbor. It is hot and Millie is due for lunch and her nap. She whines and tries to turn in her stroller. Millie's mother pauses in her conversation, peeks at the baby, and smiles reassuringly. "We'll go home real soon, Millie. I know you are tired and hungry. Give me another few minutes, okay? How about some water in the meanwhile? I bet you are thirsty." Millie stops fussing and reaches with her hand. Her mother gets a baby bottle from the stroller-bag and hands it to the child. Millie settles back into the stroller cushion and suckles on the water, content to wait a little longer.

Our world and how we understand it become shaped by our experiences and our communication with others around us. Language and communication are crucial for babies and children: What is communicated (or is not) and how it is communicated literally shapes their brain and understanding. Language includes the ways we put words together as well as the intent we invest them with. As detailed in Part 1, communication allows us to convey information about feelings, perceptions, and concepts and to ask questions about them. It allows us to express needs and ideas in requests, queries, and the sharing of thoughts and plans. It shows our understanding of others' communication through our own responses of voice, language, action, affect, and internal state.

In the vignette above, Millie communicates her distress and impatience. Her mother's language and actions reflect understanding as she verbalizes the child's discomfort and offers a temporary reprieve. Millie is still tired and hungry, but her thirst is slaked and her impatience validated. We can assume from Millie's response that she understood some of her mother's words and that she had learned through previous interactions to trust her mother to attend to her needs. The mother's sensitive response can lead us to infer that had Millie shown stronger discomfort or continued to fuss, the mother would have ended the conversation, picked the child up, offered a snack, or adjusted the stroller so Millie could sleep. Millie communicated nonverbally but her mother used language and action to impart understanding and care. The success of their communication likely followed previous positive exchanges.

Ten-month-old Ronnie's mother also stops to speak with a friend. Ronnie is hot and tired. When the conversation stretches, he whines. His mother ignores him and continues chatting. Ronnie whines louder. Getting no response, he begins crying. "Cut it out, Ronnie," his mother scolds impatiently. "Stop fussing." Ronnie tosses his hat out of the stroller. "UGH, Ronnie!" the mother bends down to pick up the cap, glares at the infant, and continues her conversation. When Ronnie continues crying, his mother thumps the stroller's handles, jarring the baby with each word. "Cut. It. Out. Can't you see I'm talking?" Ronnie startles, stops crying, and sits passively in the stroller, staring vacantly ahead.

When Ronnie stopped crying, it was not because he was soothed or understood, but because his mother's anger scared him. Too young to talk, he could not verbalize his discomfort, and his mother did not help. She neither put his experience into words nor reassured him that she would soon attend to him. Instead, her anger communicated upset at his disrupting her conversation. Ronnie's previous experience might have taught him that continued crying would lead to more anger. Maybe his mother's reaction reminded him of when her rage proved painful or terrifying. Tied into his stroller, Ronnie could not remove himself from the situation, attend to his own needs, or seek comfort elsewhere. He stopped crying even as his distress intensified, and shut down. His mother's response to his attempt to communicate his needs let him know he was a nuisance and he better stop nagging, or else.

When it comes to babies and children, the stage is exquisitely set for communication failure. Their comprehension is limited. They have no words or far fewer words than adults for describing their experience. They are still learning conversational rules and concepts such as time, order, and causation. Adults normally shoulder much of the language burden to ensure successful communication, interpreting babies' actions and reactions, narrating what the babies are doing or seem to want, verbalizing possible motivations, etc. If the interpretation matches the child's needs, communication succeeded. If the child's needs are not met, the adult likely misinterpreted the child's intent and the interaction failed.

Communication failure of itself is not a negative. Misunderstandings happen, and children can learn how to recognize and fix them: They point, repeat a word, or pull the adult to show them what they had intended. They may shake their head or cry to show frustration. Older children learn how to ask questions if they did not understand, or to rephrase what they said if others seem confused. Normal communication failure utilizes the baseline of overall successful interaction to teach repair, creative thinking, tenacity, and flexibility. However, when that baseline is missing, communication failure can lead to withdrawal, reduced interaction, and distress.

It is possible that Ronnie's mother had a bad day, was not feeling well, or for some reason was momentarily overwhelmed. If that interaction was an isolated event, it would not likely impact Ronnie's development. However, if the exchange was representative of how Ronnie's mother usually responded to his attempts to communicate needs, his language could suffer. How would he know to label body states or feelings? How would he learn to talk about things that happened and how they made him feel? Who would he tell it too? Why would he even try? How would he know that his perceptions were describable, that they mattered?

Language helps us think, compare, reason, deduct, and predict. Connections are initiated and reinforced through sharing all manner of experiences and stories. To learn language, children need to be exposed to it through the narration of their caretakers and descriptions of things, events, actions, and concepts in the child's world (Baron 1992, Berman 2004, de Boysson-Bardies 1999, Gleason & Ratner 2009, Ninio & Snow 1996). As caretakers verbalize physical states and emotional experiences, children learn to conceptualize and describe: hungry, angry, tired, warm, dry, and happy. Bedtime stories, shared conversations, and narrative of daily events weave a growing tapestry of language for a child to draw on. By kindergarten, normally developing, well-cared-for children can use language to tell stories, negotiate basic desires, share thoughts, comment, listen, and understand communicative intents (Berman 2004, Ninio & Snow 1996).

Traumatized children, however, may find communication foreign or threatening. They may fear speaking about what they want or need. They may not even know what it is. Children need support the most during overwhelm, and yet traumatizing events are often when experiences were least likely to be acknowledged and validated, let alone explained. Caregivers may be unavailable during crises (Kazak et al 2006, Kuttner 2010, Winston et al 2002), and the trauma of neglect and abuse is often ignored or deliberately denied, minimized, and distorted (Heineman 1998, Pearce & Pezzot-Pearce 1997, Putnam, 1997, Silberg, 1998, 2013, Terr 1990, Wieland 2011). Trauma alters the child's world and his/her ability to talk about it.

Trauma Narrative in Adults

Language centers are programmed to work in calm conditions. Stress disrupts the capacity to think clearly, affects information processing, formulating, and problem solving and impacts communication (van der Kolk 2014). Even relatively simple directions can be confusing or difficult to understand and/or remember under stress. Stressed persons are prone to misreading and misinterpreting what is said or needed. They may find it difficult to explain what they need and can send confusing, impatient, even unkind verbal and nonverbal signals. Stress makes people lousy communication partners.

Stress affects processing and memory. It is why doctors advise patients to bring someone along to important appointments and why people bring notes to important presentations. It is also why stressed people's sense of humor may seem dulled and what they usually find witty becomes irritating. Even moderate stress—too much to do, too little sleep—can affect language processing, let alone the overwhelm of trauma. Conceptualization, narration, and memory often change under extreme duress, which can lead to traumatic events being encoded, retrieved, and communicated differently than everyday events (Cozolino 2006, Herman 1997, Silberg 2013, van der Kolk 2014). In addition, dissociation and overwhelm can fragment traumatic events, with fragmentation further disrupting the encoding of events and making them difficult to process and share (Attias & Goodwin 1999, Levine & Maté 2010, Lehman 2005, Perry & Szalavitz 2006, Putnam 1997, Steinberg & Schnall 2000).

Trauma can defy words. People who survived traumatic events often say things like "words can't describe it," "it was beyond words," or "I can't find the words to explain it." These expressions depict how un-word-able trauma can feel. Survivors frequently find it difficult to explain how they felt, how they knew what they know, and why they reacted the way they did. They may not fully comprehend how things unfolded or how to describe it. "If you weren't there, you wouldn't understand," they may say, "I wasn't thinking, I just acted," or "I don't know how I got from A to B, it just happened."

Affect is an integral part of communication, too. Pleasant emotions like joy, love, and connection can heighten perception, communication, wit, processing, and memory, while unpleasant emotions like terror, helplessness, and despair can have the opposite effect. When people are flooded by difficult emotions, they may be less able to understand other people and less likely to be understood. They may overreact (e.g. panic) or underreact (i.e. detach, shut down, dissociate), with both extremes affecting the ability to extract and process information. Cynicism, satire, and metaphor require simultaneous processing of both literal meanings and implied intention, but overwhelmed people do not do well reading between the lines.

Trauma evokes strong emotions: fear, worry, terror, pain, rage, confusion, horror, helplessness, despair, conflict, guilt, and many more. These feelings can persist when the person feels unable to put words to what happened or feels others do not understand, leaving survivors panicked and irritable, angry, scattered, and confused. Posttraumatic narrative can be incoherent and inconsistent. Some people may seem overly dramatic or exaggerating while others may narrate their experiences in a detached way that leads others to think they were unaffected, are lying, or do not care (Herman 1997, van der Kolk 2014). When traumatized persons 'make no sense' or 'do not have expected feelings,' others may find it difficult to be empathetic. Traumatized people themselves may not feel connected to what happened or to themselves. Under normal circumstances, being able to recognize, differentiate, name, and understand affect allows us to feel connected to ourselves and to other people and reinforces successful communication. When feelings are so overwhelming that what they bring up is incomprehensible and feels impossible to explain, ordinary words lose power. Connection and language fail.

Trauma isolates and disrupts communication. Maybe not surprisingly, it is often the sharing and finding words to communicate it that help heal and assist in making sense of what was beyond words (Herman 1997). Trauma work encompasses more than 'talk therapy.' The value of body therapies and working through the physiological aspects of trauma is increasingly appreciated (Levine & Kline 2007, van der Kolk 2014). Nevertheless, putting one's experience in words, being heard and understood, remains part of trauma recovery. Language facilitates the integration of traumatic events into the tapestry of life and into one's story. In Herman's words, it is the "testifying that brings back the victim's voice" (Herman 1997).

The Importance of Context and Pre-Trauma Skills

When adults struggle to deal with traumatic experiences, they do so with some understanding of the world and with language to draw from. Adults may know— at least cognitively—that though someone harmed them, it does not mean that the whole world turned unsafe. They have experience with managing everyday stressors, conflict, and disappointment, along with some sense of calm, relaxation, and focusing. Most adults are able to understand—or at least identify— other people's confusing or irrational behaviors. They can draw on connections and attachment to others to get through. They know bad things can end.

Even under duress, adults may have some context for what happened—they may be in terrible pain being treated after a car accident, but they know what an accident is and that the doctors are trying to help. An injured person may know that help is likely to come, where they might go for support, that some things are illegal and who to report them to. They understand that natural disasters are outside their control (i.e. not their fault). Using their world knowledge, adults can draw comparisons to try and identify at least some of how they feel. They might say "I was more terrified than I have ever been before," or "this was worse than a thousand wasp-stings," or "I felt so alone!" They have perspective and life knowledge with which to understand and verbalize some of what they experience.

Yet even with world knowledge and a well-developed language, trauma can be very difficult to find the words for. Adults often struggle to recall some aspects of what happened while at the same time being flooded by other aspects of it (Herman 1997, Levine & Maté 2010, Wallin 2007, van der Hart et al 2006, van der Kolk 2014). They may feel confused or that even if they tried to explain, no one would understand. Some feel that no words would work and that something fundamental in them was changed by the trauma, that there is no describing what they endured.

Healing often includes reaffirming connections to other people and using life experiences before the trauma as anchor. People may remember places they felt safe in—physically and otherwise—and 'visualize' those safe places to reorient when trauma memories overwhelm. They may work to release the trauma stored in their bodies so that calm can be restored. Traumatized adults might journal or find a common language with others who endured similar hardship. They can tell their story and find hope (Cozolino 2014, Herman 1997, Schwartz 2000, Schore 2012, van der Hart et al 2006, van der Kolk 2014).

Nothing to Compare to—Early Trauma and Lack of Baseline Skills

Verbalizing trauma can be difficult for people who have mature language skills and an understanding of the world. How much more difficult for children, who have yet to acquire language and who lack a full concept of the world? As a group, children have less access to emotional regulation, a narrow base of life experience, and a limited understanding of context or options. A loud thunderclap may startle an adult, but it can terrify a young child who does not know what it is, what it means, or what would happen next. Because physiological regulation is still emerging in children, they often rely on others to help them regulate from panic and learn what is or is not life-threatening (Cozolino 2006, Schore 2001).

Children are intrinsically vulnerable. They can rarely remove themselves from a scary situation and may not be aware of the possibility of leaving even when it is there. They may be unable to identify that they are getting upset or scared, let alone explain what scared them. When language is either unavailable or inadequate to describe reality—let alone in posttraumatic states when language centers are suppressed—the child is left with "mute hopelessness about the possibility of communicating. . . . [W]ords are both too powerful and completely useless" (Strong 1999, p. 44).

The impact of trauma on children's connection and communication is especially devastating because children develop attachment and language at the same time. A parent's 'word' for something—an object, feeling, event—becomes the child's understanding for that thing. What a caregiver says (or does not say) is interwoven into the assumptions and beliefs a child has about the world. What an adult communicates becomes the child's reality. Without much life experience to compare to, trauma can influence how a child understands meaning in ways that affects not only trauma-related material but other interactions as well.

For children, trauma may not be something outside the scope of expectation: If it happened, it may well happen again; and so any small reminder of it can become an omen of imminent overwhelm. If trauma indeed repeats (as is often the case in maltreatment), there may be little 'normal' to contrast trauma with. If trauma is likely in everyday interactions, children automatically apply posttraumatic and dissociative reactions (e.g. numbing, re-experiencing), reinforcing a cycle of anxiety, reactivity, and overwhelm.

Ami's teacher could not figure out why the child froze anytime someone ran in the hallway. "It is just a kid running!" she puzzled. "They're not supposed to run in the hallway, but it is not like something bad is happening." To Ami, however, the sound of running indicated danger, someone trying to escape. Her limited repertoire dictated her interpretation, and because she froze at the first sound of running, her belief—and dissociation—became reinforced.

Children whose lives were overall safe, with sensitive caregivers who helped them regulate distress, can use supportive experience to fall back on after overwhelm, especially if they have a healthy baseline of language and communication skills. This is not the case for children whose upbringing was difficult. This is not the case for those whose communication skills are compromised by language/learning issues, autism and developmental delay, deafness, stuttering, attention deficits, and emotional difficulties. Disabilities not only increase a child's risk for maltreatment and trauma (Benedict et al 1990, Crosse et al 1993, Goldson 1998, Hershkowitz et al 2007, Sullivan et al 1987, Sullivan & Knutson 1998, 2000), but they place the child at a disadvantage in comprehending, processing, and narrating what happened to them, compounding the child's overwhelm and limiting people's ability to help.

Very young children, children with disabilities, and children who experience maltreatment may have a narrow or even paradoxical comprehension of concepts. Even if the child tries to verbalize his or her experience, others might misunderstand, because their assumption about the meaning of a concept is different. Such miscommunication can leave a child feeling confused and unheard, further reinforcing helplessness and inability to get help.

Every time Miriam's uncle came to visit, her momma would call her and announce: "Miriam, your favorite uncle is here! Aren't you happy to see him?" That uncle would often take Miriam on 'special trips' which inevitably meant confusing and painful things that scared her but she was told she liked . . . For four-year-old Miriam, "favorite" meant "the one who hurts," and being happy to see someone meant feeling afraid, anxious, and trapped. When a neighbor asked Miriam about her uncle's visit, the child murmured, "I was happy to see him." When the preschool teacher asked who the man who came to pick her up from school was, Miriam whispered: "My favorite uncle." She tried to communicate, but instead of getting help and being protected, Miriam received reactions that indicated people thought she should spend even more time with her uncle.

When Communication Itself Is Stressful, Confusing, and Frightening

Leigh was rescued by police when they raided the 'crack house' his mother and her boyfriend lived in. Both adults were under the influence when police found the one-year-old in a crib. He was undernourished and had sores on his bottom from unchanged diapers. His mother sported bruises, possibly from domestic violence. Leigh's X-rays showed evidence of radial fracture of his arm and what looked like healed rib fractures. Child Protection Services placed him in a foster-family, where suspicions of autism were raised because the child did not make eye contact and was like a 'sack of potatoes' when he was picked up. Leigh did not respond to his name and often turned away rather than toward his foster-mother. He could cry for hours in a keening voice that the foster-mother admitted "drove her up the walls." Nothing consoled him. Picking him up only made it worse.

When the communication children are exposed to is loud, scary, and violent, they might find the sound of people frightening. Needing adults to care for them but simultaneously feeling terrified of contact, children may not know what to do or how to make use of comfort when it is offered. Did Leigh's parents talk to him? Did they call him by name? What did it mean to him when they did? What if being addressed meant pain? If making eye contact enrages caregivers, children learn to avert their eyes. They may not learn that it is part of how people are expected to relate.

For children who endured care by neglectful, abusive, mentally ill, addicted (and unpredictable) persons, communication can be bewildering and scary. Children may not know how to respond to (or initiate) social exchanges, turn-take, or listen. They may not recognize that a certain discomfort means 'hungry' and another 'tired.' To them discomfort may be an undifferentiated and unpredictable pain that they do not understand or know how to tell someone about to soothe it. Even after their circumstances change, some children do not know how to communicate needs or what is expected. If asked, "Are you hungry?" they may eat even if full because they believe they must. They might say "no" even though they are hungry because they don't know what to make of the question or believe they should refuse. They might become afraid, if being asked a question had meant punishment and pain.

Lack of comprehension compounds the overwhelm that is inherent to trauma. Children may not know what to expect, especially if painful things happened without warning or apparent cause. Maltreatment does not come with sensitive explanations. Abusive caregivers do not say to a child: "I see that you are feeling really angry at me because you need me to help you but you feel frightened every time I enter the room because I might beat you up so you don't know what to do about my proximity . . ." Neglectful caregivers do not narrate: "I know you are very hungry and that you really need me to go get you more food. I know you must be confused why I am not coming to comfort you and just turn my back on you and watch TV." Not only are maltreatment experiences rarely discussed, they are often deliberately denied or distorted (Heineman 1998, Putnam 1997, Schwartz 2000, Silberg 1998, 2013).

If a caregiver laughs at a child's terror, a child may confuse 'funny' with scary. They may believe that when people laugh, one should be scared. If a caregiver slaps the child out of the blue and says: "What are you crying about?" or "Look what you made me do!"—what is the child to understand? Why is she crying? What did she do? To maltreated children, being noticed might mean pain, being called by one's name might mean to expect a beating, a grin could mean feeling terrified. Caregivers do not have to be consistently cruel or neglectful to confuse a child's understanding of communication. Many traumatized children have caregivers who sometimes talk to them, cuddle them, and care for them but at other times turn frightening, mocking, and confusing. For such children, being talked to can mean comfort or it can mean pain, and they may have little way to predict—let alone control—whether the attention will bring calm or overwhelm. How would their communication not suffer?

Traumatized children can be wary, odd, or inappropriate communicators. They may not follow directions or express emotions well, they may not "use their words" or know how to describe what they are experiencing. What they do describe can be confusing or misunderstood because of the context they derive it from (e.g. Miriam and her 'favorite' uncle). Adults usually attempt to interpret children's communications, but it can be difficult to know what to make of the reactions of a child who speaks a 'relational language' that does not make sense to us. It is distressing to have a child cry when we smile at them, scream louder when we try to comfort her, or smear feces on the wall during his birthday party . . .

The baseline for communicating perceptions, feelings, body states, thoughts, and questions can be missing in maltreated children, and it does not miraculously appear when care is offered. When they 'misbehave,' their communications are often interpreted as 'bad,' manipulative, autistic, antisocial, aggressive, uncaring, and cruel. If they are shamed or punished, their assumptions about the world's unfairness becomes reinforced. Misunderstandings are difficult for anyone and are even more so for traumatized children, who don't know how to respond well to failed interactions. They may 'zone out' and stop communicating, or 'talk back' and become aggressive, hurtful, and "unreasonably argumentative." The stage is often set for dissonance, anger, and distance between the child and others to increase.

While they may not be particularly effective in healthy communications, maltreated children are nevertheless powerful communicators: Misunderstandings and misbehaviors can in fact be a window into the children's 'language of trauma'—their experiences and needs. By remaining sensitive to how the child responds and reacts, and what aspects of communication are impacted by trauma, we can help reduce miscommunication and offer grounding and reparative narratives to help the child's language of relating expand.

8 Trauma's Impact on Attention and Learning

Attention and Learning

Listening is an active process that requires allocation of energies so one can detect, discriminate, identify, and comprehend (Heymann 2010). Listening and learning require attention: We cannot learn if we are unconscious, checked out, or dissociated or are actively shutting down what is taking place because we find it overwhelming. Indeed, many maltreated children are diagnosed with attention issues and language/learning issues and are more likely to need special education settings (Beverly et al 2008, Cole et al 2005, Putnam 1997, Fox et al 1988, Kurtz et al 1993, Martin & Dombrowski 2008, Pearce & Pezzot-Pearce 1997, Scherr 2007, Silberg 1998, Waters 2005, Wodarski et al 1990, Yehuda 2004, 2005).

The relationship between trauma and attention is complex. In some children, attention issues are due to hypervigilance and/or dissociation: They are unable to attend because they are too anxious or too shut down to remain engaged. Their posttraumatic fluctuations in presentation can lead to a misdiagnosis of attention-deficit hyperactivity disorder (ADD/ADHD). Other children may have a predisposition for attention deficits that trauma exacerbates. Children with attention deficits are at high risk for maltreatment (Briscoe-Smith & Hinshaw 2006, Fuller-Thomson et al 2014, Goldson 1998, Knutson & Sullivan 1993, Nadeau & Nolin 2013) and are vulnerable to overwhelm even without maltreatment, due to how attention deficits bring frequent failure, confusion, and frustration. Whether a child's inattention is from primary ADD/ADHD, due to worsening of attention deficits following trauma, or reflects posttraumatic and dissociative coping, a child who cannot attend well will not be able to learn to his/her potential.

Attention itself is a complex process. Different levels and types of attentiveness connect with and are influenced by aspects of awareness and perception, and the interplay of these factors serves to reinforce or dampen attention and engagement. Interest interacts closely with attention: An interested listener is better positioned to extract meaning and nuances from an interaction. Indeed, the processing of intent, ambiguity, humor, symbolic language, and metaphor all require attention (Ninio & Snow 1996). Emotional connection helps interest. A conversation one feels emotionally connected to is more likely to keep one's attention. Both interest and connection help us acquire and store new information. It is why optimal conditions for learning are when students are interested, actively engaged, and available to attend (e.g. not hungry, tired, or physically uncomfortable).

Attention under Stress

Comfortable engagement enhances attention and learning, but discomfort and stress dampen processing and distract from learning and comprehending. Stress changes the quality of focus as the body narrows perceptions and attention to what can ensure immediate survival (van der Kolk 2014). Blood gets pumped to the extremities, pupils dilate to receive more light, adrenaline floods the body, hearing acuity to sounds may heighten while the processing of linguistic information gets suppressed—the opposite of calm focus that is required for new learning (Scaer 2014, van der Kolk 2014). Though one can learn to react reflexively under stress (think: military training), assimilation of new information is reduced by stress even when motivation to attend is high. A newly diagnosed patient may be intensely interested in what the doctor has to say, yet people are advised to bring someone along to important medical appointments: The stress involved in life-altering information can override language processing and reduce the quality of listening, processing, and remembering.

It makes sense that learning will take a back seat to survival: Identifying cries of warning that warrant immediate response is crucial in danger, but the processing of new concepts, explanations, and views is not a priority when one is trying to stay alive. Academics or definitions of new words are not foremost on your mind as you are trying to escape an avalanche or outrun a tiger. You are not likely to enjoy a weather pun or a lecture about the preferred habitat of tigers. Though you may hear the voice of the person you have been on the phone with or called for help, you probably won't be responding to subtle social cues or content questions: Your resources are fully occupied in not being buried alive or becoming lunch.

Most incidences of avalanche escape or tiger fleeing resolve rapidly (one way or the other . . .), and if safety is restored, your body can slowly calm enough to allow you to process what just took place. That is when language comes in, after the danger passes, and you can reflect on what took place and share it with others. It is only when safe that you will be able—even feel compelled—to recount the fear, try to piece together how it happened, where the snow or tiger came from, what and how you felt when you noticed a blurry danger hurling toward you, how you reacted (and even how annoyed you were that the person on the phone kept prattling about who knows what instead of realizing you were franticly escaping smothering or mauling). This kind of processing is important—it is often only after it takes place and you 'get it out of your system' that your body calms so attention to other things resumes and mundane life feels real again (Herman 1997, Levine & Maté 2010, van der Kolk 2014). However, if overwhelming stress remains ongoing or unprocessed, the ability to return to calm attentiveness, listening, and learning is stalled (Scaer 2014, Siegel 2012, van der Kolk 2014).

Even adults with mature attending skills find it difficult to listen and process under duress, let alone children whose abilities are still developing—even more so for those children experiencing chronic stress and who may lack a physiological baseline for what calm attention and listening can be like (Cozolino 2014, van der Kolk 2005). Maltreatment does not produce good listeners, and as a group, traumatized children often struggle with attending (Silberg 2013, Yehuda 2004, 2005, 2011). They may listen inconsistently: remembering parts of the instruction but not well enough to succeed. They may not know how to differentiate what is or is not important. Living in survival mode (whether due to ongoing trauma or posttraumatic activation) renders them unable to allocate sufficient attention to learning and assimilating new information—they are too busy trying to outrun avalanches and tigers.

Both at school and at home, traumatized children are required to attend and listen, yet are doing so with systems that are neurologically suboptimally available for effective learning. If stress continues, their brains might become even less available for learning. Neuronal complexity grows best where it is reinforced (Gaensbauer 2011, Schore 2001, 2012, Siegel 2012). Well-cared-for, nontraumatized children spend most waking hours in calm attentive curiosity geared for learning. The areas of the brain involved in attending, listening, assimilating, processing, integrating, and retrieving information get plenty of use and become increasingly efficient at doing so. Children who are available for learning become better learners. They can utilize learning opportunities to assemble, process, associate, retrieve, and use information.

This is not the case for children who are less available for learning. Whether due to hypervigilance or shutting down, children who cannot attend well become less efficient learners. Learning opportunities can be harder for them to take advantage of. They may require more repetitions in more contexts to process and associate new information with things already learned, because stress also impacts brain areas responsible for memory organization and accessibility (i.e. the limbic system, hippocampus) (Stien & Kendall 2004, van der Kolk 2014). This makes knowledge less accessible while trauma reminders remain easily triggered. Overwhelmed children struggle to maintain attention, with inconsistent listening and spotty learning (Silberg 2013, Yehuda 2011).

Listening—Too Much, Too Little, All at Once and Not at All

Listening goes well beyond detecting a sound or hearing something being said; it requires attending to and integrating what is heard with additional clues (e.g. emotional, visual, sensory) that can assist in processing. To listen well, one needs to focus on what needs to be listened to and dampen attention to background noises, along with the flexibility to quickly shift that focus (e.g. attend to one speaker, then the other) (Bellis 2002, Heymann 2010).

Because listening is impacted by trauma, chronic traumatization can affect the development of listening skills. Children who are hypervigilant cannot focus on a teacher's voice or the words of a caregiver because they treat everything around them as potential danger. Instruction gets drowned by the child's occupation with everything but—environmental noises, other people's footsteps, the sound of their own breathing, the hum of an air-conditioner, or as they generally brace for scary sounds yet to come. Traumatized children can be hypervigilant in what seems to be a calm classroom or a safe home (Levine & Kline 2007, Perry & Szalavitz 2006, Silberg 2013, Wieland 2011). Their anxious alertness renders them unavailable to learning.

Shut-down children do not listen either. They may not feel safe remaining attentive because they fear to hear things that would trigger flooding of helplessness and terror (Gomez 2012, Silberg 2013, Wieland 2011). Even if what is said interests them, they may be too overwhelmed to take chances. They miss opportunities for comfort, curiosity, and fun as they turn attention off and snail in. Some traumatized children may use hypervigilance or numbing as their main strategy of coping, but many oscillate, shifting from attending to everything and becoming flooded, to shutting down and shutting off (Waters 2005, Silberg 2013, Wieland 2011). They may listen intermittently and get snippets of information, but their listening is not learning oriented.

To listen for learning involves noting meaningful variations and ignoring unimportant ones. A change in a speaker's tone may shift the meaning of "she is *not* here" to "she is not *here*" while other tone variations may not change meaning. Listening requires discriminating between close sounds: Was the direction "wait" or "paste"? Did the parent say, "You can" or "you can't"? Listening includes attending to the words as well as to the context in which they are spoken. It requires identifying when context dictates meaning (e.g. "she's down in the dumps").

A traumatized child who is focused on the teacher's tone or facial expressions (e.g. to watch for anger) or her hands (e.g. if they learned to be wary of those) can miss the content of what she is saying. Their hypervigilance can extend to people who never harmed them. Faces, hands, and tones may be all they know to attend to. Difficulties listening exact more than an academic price; it leaves the child less experienced with attending and managing interpersonal interactions, too. Reducing children's need for dissociation and increasing their internal sense of safety is paramount for improving listening and enabling learning.

"Like a 24-Hour Sonar"—Leah: When Overwhelm Overrides Awareness

Leah grew up under fire, literally. From age four to six, her hometown was frequently subject to missile and rocket fire. Her life revolved around shrill alarms, running to find shelter, and the detritus of explosions. Nights were punctuated with sirens and more rushing to shelter. Preschool, home routines, and play all could be disrupted at any moment. Then Leah's father had a job offer overseas, and the family moved to the US.

Leah had been toilet trained by two and a half, but she began to wet her bed again when her family lived in the war zone. She had developed rigid routines, too: wearing only certain pajamas and donning only sneakers "to run fast." She feared going to bed at night and worried that a rocket would fall on her like it did on a neighbor. Even after the family moved to New York and away from missiles, Leah still woke her parents with night terrors. Her rigidity continued. Everything had to be done in a particular order or Leah would have a meltdown: her place setting, which towel she got to use, how her mother combed her hair. She had frequent and sometimes violent tantrums at home, some of which she claimed to not remember. Leah had been diagnosed with ADHD, anxiety, sensory integration, and an eye to possible obsessive compulsive disorder.

Leah's family arrived in New York in time for her to start first grade. She was jumpy and impulsive at school, rarely waited her turn, called out answers prematurely, and rushed through assignments with many mistakes (and meltdowns). The teachers were empathic—knowing Leah was learning a new language and adjusting to new routines and longer school days. The school had experience with transplanted students. Staff expected children to need time to acclimate, and tolerated initial difficulties with concentrating. Leah, however, did not seem to acclimate and an increase in ADHD medication did not help. Her abilities, concentration, and behavior lagged significantly behind those of other new students and were low in her first language, too. She was referred to me for speech-language therapy.

Leah displayed many symptoms usually associated with ADHD: impulsiveness, irritability, fidgeting, and distractibility. Hypervigilance in children can look very much the same. Leah took fidgeting to a whole new level. Some part of her was always moving in one way or another: her head, her eyes, her legs, her mouth, her hands. She was restless even when involved with things she loved, like watching videos. She seemed perpetually poised to bolt, kicking and jerking even in her sleep. "She is like a 24-hour sonar," her mother stated. "At least she's no longer sleepwalking," she added. The year before, the family had to install high latches and bells on doors to keep the girl from wandering out at night.

Leah's school was adept at utilizing ADHD management tools: schedule prompts, points and stars for attending and completing tasks, a squeeze-ball for letting out the *fidgets, frequent breaks. Nothing worked well enough. Sitting with her back to the classroom door, Leah constantly turned; facing the door, she would constantly monitor passersby. She "disintegrated" whenever someone ran in the hallway. Ambulance sirens reduced her to sobbing. She had to be taken home after the first fire drill and the child refused school for days following. "This one is wound very tight," the teacher sighed. "Her eyes look open but they are shut to learning. This kid is not really here."*

Focusing and Shifting Focus—the Relative Importance of Everything

Selective attention is part of listening. In order to listen to what the teacher is saying, we need to also *not* listen to other things. The teacher's words take precedence over the feeling of one's seat in the chair, the smell from the cafeteria, the shaft of light on the floor, the whispering of peers behind you, the scraping of a chair someplace in the room. All these get perceived and may register somewhere in awareness, but it is background. The focus remains the teacher, the information, the task at hand.

Good listening requires focus, but also the ability to shift focus quickly and flexibly between what is 'figure' and what is 'ground.' We can be on the phone and shift to answer a child's question or let someone know the dryer is done. We can momentarily eavesdrop on the conversation of the people at a nearby restaurant table by shifting focus so their voices become foreground instead of the discussion at our table. This fluid shifting is very different than the alarm of danger where stress floods the body and focus scatters to scan any stimuli as potentially lifesaving or life endangering. It is different than the hyperfocused 'tunnel vision' where all but what supports survival is disregarded (e.g. not feeling the pain of injuries, 'not seeing' what is happening around one). Hypervigilance and hyperfocus can be lifesaving in a brief emergency but exact a high price in exhaustion, health, and development if maintained (Felitti et al 1998, Kendall-Tackett 2002, Nijenhuis 2004, Scaer 2014, van der Kolk 2014).

Stress activates detection and identification (e.g. is there danger? What is coming?) but suppresses comprehension, integration, and processing (van der Kolk 2014). Hypervigilant children may want to listen to a story but be constantly pulled to attend to a cough in another room, the beep of a distant car, the breathing of a peer. When these children also have limited language and world knowledge, they might not have the context and concepts for identifying and recognizing some sounds as neutral, remaining vigilant for harm. The best narrative and teaching cannot reach a child who is too activated to listen, and requiring a child to 'pay attention' does not help. What can help is awareness of the impact of stress on listening and understanding and identifying hypervigilance (or shutting down), and helping children get grounded and better regulated. Only then can we help children build a foundation for improved attending (see Part 5).

Listening for Information—When Nothing Makes Sense, How Does One Make Sense of Anything?

Children's listening evolves as it helps them make sense of the world around them. Maltreated children may not know that listening can be helpful. Severely neglected children may not realize that when someone talks, information is imparted. If talking takes place 'over their heads' as caregivers speak to each other but very little of their talk is child directed, children will not learn that listening is helpful (Miller 2005). Abused children may learn that it is better not to listen (Gaensbauer 2011).

Listening is taught with the earliest interactions. When we respond to a baby's sounds and movements, we reinforce that listening has meaning—you do something, and another person notices and understands it. We teach listening when we narrate a baby's discomfort and soothe it: Our words accompany care and the baby listens (Cozolino 2006, 2014). When previous interactions taught a baby that words mean comfort, she calms down when we say: "Let's go home so I can change your diaper." The toddler learns that words have power when he says "wet" and we do something about it. Listening develops through the experience of being talked to and listened to. Without it, babies do not know to listen. They may hear and not respond. They may respond but not attend.

Many traumatized children have had some experience with listening and being listened to, yet also experienced traumatizing realities that were (or felt) unattended to. Abusive parents rarely listen to the child's experience when they harm the child. They often ignore, minimize, or distort it. Overwhelmed parents may not realize that the child is hurting, upset, or terrified. Children internalize that they are not someone worth listening to. They may learn that they must listen all the time and that no amount of listening prevents more hurting or explains the incomprehensible. What does "you made me do it" or "see what you've done?" mean when you have no idea what you did or how it is related to what has happened? Does listening even matter if what takes place does not make sense? What does "happy now?" mean when you are sad? What does it mean when you respond "No" and get laughed at, ignored, or hurt anyway? If listening does not work, children might stop trying to do it, and when they turn off listening, they miss opportunities to learn how to listen and process information.

Auditory processing basically means what we do with what we hear. A child who does not attend or retain auditory information will not be able to comprehend it well or store it effectively for later retrieval. Yet we assume auditory processing abilities whenever we ask children to follow directions, comprehend stories, or determine what a question was about; whenever we expect them to recall facts, formulate opinions, or understand riddles, inferences, and abstractions.

Dissociation affects listening and processing: You cannot be both shut down and engaged. Even when children manage to attend, trauma reminders that bring on periods of dissociation can result in fragments of instruction that then do not add up or make sense (Silberg 2013, Wieland 2011). Children may make mistakes and feel misunderstood or realize that what they heard does not make sense and feel stupid because others seem to get it. If scolded or told that they are not trying hard enough, children might decide that listening is not worth the trouble, makes them feel bad, or is scary.

"Book-Blank Kid"—Marcus: Dyslexia, Auditory Processing, or Dissociation?

Marcus' language/learning issues manifested especially in auditory and literacy activities. The eight-year-old frequently 'zoned out' in class, but even when he seemed to be listening, he made many errors: copied the wrong words, did the wrong page, completely missed the point of a story. The teachers wondered about 'dyslexia' and 'attention deficit,' and the school psychologist suspected an auditory processing disorder.

Filling in for another professional, it was the second half of the school year by the time I first met Marcus. The second grader struggled with reading. Even very easy sight-word books made him anxious. He mostly guessed, and when he got things wrong he refused to try again. He did not like listening to stories, either. Soft-spoken and gentle, Marcus did not explode, hit other kids, or yell. He imploded. Stopped responding, became blank, stared. During literacy time, Marcus would sit at his chair without looking at the book on his desk. He would not choose a book and if the teacher chose one for him, he did not fuss, just did not look at it. If read to, he still zoned out.

The teacher liked Marcus but his behavior drove her nuts. "He is very manipulative about it," she complained. "Stubborn as a mule . . . If he decides not to do something, you can promise or threaten, and he won't do it, just stand there until I give up or time runs out." What added to the teacher's frustration was how Marcus could be "a totally different kid" in some other classes. The gym teacher praised the boy for his focus and teamwork. The art teacher gushed over his creative application. "It is like he is allergic to literacy," the classroom teacher sighed. "As long as it does not involve reading or writing, he is in school heaven. Add a book, and he checks out. Dyslexia or not, this is one book-blank kid!"

Teachers' observations are often invaluable descriptors of children, so I always listen. Some children with dyslexia avoid written materials like the plague, but they may still enjoy listening to stories. Children with auditory processing disorder often enjoy picture books and have difficulties in many listening settings. Something else or something more was going on with Marcus. He enjoyed 'magic messages' in code pages, reproduced complicated strings of symbols from memory, could follow directions in gym, art, and science. Yet he struggled with even simple questions about easy stories.

Information from the teacher of Marcus' older brother was illuminating. It seemed that Marcus' mother left an abusive situation when Marcus was in kindergarten.

For a time she and the kids lived with the mother's grand-aunt, who watched the children when the mother worked nights. Apparently Marcus' brother disclosed abuse by the relative. Child services got involved and both boys were found with bruises on the clothes-covered areas of their bodies. They were briefly in foster-care until the mother was cleared of charges and found secure housing: It was the grand-aunt who tormented the boys. After the mother left for work, the older woman would declare "story time" and read the boys "bad stories" from newspapers about harm to children. She would quiz the children and pinch them viciously, threatening that their mother would "fall down dead" if they told . . . No surprise Marcus hated anything to do with 'stories', books, or reading. No wonder he shut down whenever he was asked to listen to one or remember what it was about.

We revisit Marcus in Chapter 16, but whatever the situation his mother fled from, we can assume that the boy experienced stress even before moving to live with the grand-aunt and her inescapable torment. Telling meant losing his mother, and for little Marcus, listening to stories became synonymous with being scared and hurt. He stopped listening. At school, the very term "story time" was a trigger, as were books and printed pages. The direction to "sit down and listen" reminded him of stories that were terrifying. He could not escape the classroom. He could not escape the repeated introduction of books, reading, and writing by the teachers, by me . . . We were trying to teach him the very things that frightened him. No one raised a hand or voice to him at school, but it had to be confusing to have people who seemed to care do things that scare. How can reading be a good thing when it is a bad thing with bad stories? Listening did not make sense, but Marcus kept being asked to do it. The only remedy he knew was to shut down.

9 Trauma's Impact on Children's Vocabulary and Semantics

Language competency—how well one is able to comprehend meaning and convey it—is often associated with vocabulary, and lexical ability has been correlated with verbal IQ and overall cognitive ability (Gleason & Ratner 2009). Though vocabulary is not a full language measure, it represents the 'cache' of semantic items in one's language, including labels for persons, places, things, and actions and descriptors such as adjectives, adverbs, prepositions, temporal, sequential, and numerical words. Our lexicon (aka vocabulary) contains the words with which we put sentences together and express varied meanings.

Young children acquire vocabulary from words used by their caregivers. Infants don't have preconceived ideas about words—they don't even know that words exist. It is the context and content in which words are used that help children derive meaning (Baron 1992, Berman 2004, de Boysson-Bardies 1999, Ninio & Snow 1996). Words that are presented frequently, in varied sentences and in a context that is relevant to the child, are more likely to be acquired than words that are used rarely or are irrelevant to the child. Caregivers shape meaning: The meaning a caregiver gives something, verbally or through action, intonation, and consequence, is the meaning the child will learn.

Children's exposure affects their development. Language will not develop without exposure, and poor exposure such as in neglect, leads to limited cognitive and language capabilities (Albers et al 2005, Beverly et al 2008, Bowlby 1997, Cohen 2001, Cozolino 2006, Cross 2004, De Bellis 2005, Hildyard & Wolfe 2002, Hough & Kaczmarek 2011, Miller 2005, Milot et al 2010). Stress also affects brain growth and cognitive potential, and traumatized children are at higher risk for language issues than nontraumatized children and have lexical and semantic difficulties as part of difficulties with language knowledge and use (Cozolino 2014, Pearce & Pezzot-Pearce 1997, Putnam 1997, Siegel 2012, Silberg 1998, van der Kolk 2014, Yehuda 2004, 2005, 2011).

Expressive and Receptive Language

Receptive language represents the language one is able to comprehend and respond to, while expressive language represents one's use of language when communicating. Receptive and expressive lexicons are highly correlated but not necessarily identical. Many people have larger receptive vocabularies than expressive vocabularies, and it is common for people to 'know' (i.e. recognize and comprehend) many words they read or listen to but never use (Berman 2004, Gleason & Ratner 2009). Exposure to stories and literacy plays an important role in vocabulary expansion. It enriches connection, language, and semantic growth well before independent reading is achieved and continues to expand vocabularies throughout life. Children who are read to tend to have larger receptive vocabularies and better listening and processing skills (Gleason & Ratner 2009, Heymann 2010, Landry et al 2006b).

Maltreatment poses a risk for language development. As a group, maltreated children use fewer lexical items (fewer different words) and can label less lexical items than well-cared-for peers (De Bellis 2005, Kurtz et al 1993, Pearce & Pezzot-Pearce 1997, Putnam 1997). Having a limited semantic cache also means a smaller store of words to draw on for expression. Of all maltreated children, the vocabularies of neglected children tend to be the most affected (Albers et al 2005, Miller 2005). Both receptive and expressive vocabularies suffer in children who had little experience with interaction (e.g. orphanages) or whose interactions were limited to directive and repetitive utterances ("Cut it out!" "Come here," "Shut up!" "Here," "Stop fussing," "Give it to me!"). Children from homes where caregivers are overwhelmed (e.g. overworked or stressed, disabled, homeless) are also at risk for having smaller vocabularies (Levendosky et al 2003, Milot et al 2010, Nabors et al 2004).

Exposure is not the only factor in vocabulary growth. Vocabularies of traumatized children who have plenty of opportunities for interaction can be affected, too, by how stress shuts down listening and learning. Trauma and posttraumatic overwhelm can make it difficult for children to attend to interactions and less able to process and store new vocabulary (see Chapter 8). Trauma itself can thwart comprehension if it leads to scary associations and confusing meanings (e.g. Millie's 'favorite' uncle), which can inhibit inquiry and exploration.

As part of normal development, children often 'try out' new words or phrases, and adults' reactions helps them see whether they 'got it right' or not (Baron 1992, Berman 2004, Dromi 1987). If well-treated children make an error using a new word, they usually receive affectionate correction or rephrasing. Correct use often elicits praise and delight. Both reactions reinforce the child's motivation to continue to test new words. Maltreated children may not receive encouragement to experiment or be given many opportunities to narrate their experiences. Some do not know how to express themselves. Some may worry that talking can lead to bad things or about the consequence of erring. Children who are warned to "not tell" (e.g. about abuse, domestic violence, parental addiction) may limit speaking, lest something slip. Some get so anxious about talking that they stop speaking altogether in certain situations (e.g. certain cases of 'selective mutism').

Even without threats, maltreated children can be wary of mistakes. They might have been made to feel 'stupid' for misunderstanding, which discourages them from asking about or testing new words and phrases.

Not all traumatized children are maltreated, but trauma itself can make expressing oneself difficult (Herman 1997). Medically traumatized children describe feeling like their experiences "had no words," could not be put into words, and like words were not enough to explain them. Some felt that words would hurt their caregivers (e.g. they'd get upset by a child's expression of despair or pain) and so stopped trying to find ways to explain (Carlsson et al 2008, Carter 2002, Drew 2007). Some do not have the energy to do so. Chronic pain can be too occupying to allow learning, and malaise and medications' side effects can make attending difficult (Fuemmeler et al 2002, Gil et al 1991, Kazak et al 2006, Kuttner 2010, Stafstrom et al 2002, Varni et al 1996). Like other overwhelmed children, medically traumatized children may be less available to process new information and/or retrieve vocabulary they already have.

Just like in many other skills, less use can translate to less development. The ramifications of limited language use (from less exposure, reduced opportunity, dissociation, confusion, fear, restricted growth, preoccupation, etc.) in children are serious. Language requires ongoing, flexible, and creative use to develop, and disruption during early childhood can have lasting effects. While all language domains can be affected by trauma, some aspects of vocabulary and semantics appear especially vulnerable to chronic overwhelm. The following sections will detail them and explore possible reasons why.

'Body State' and Emotive Vocabulary

Traumatized children tend to use less body-state words such as hungry, tired, thirsty, hurting, or satisfied and less emotive vocabulary (Pearce & Pezzot-Pearce 1997, Putnam 1997, Silberg 1998, Yehuda 2005, 2011). Their 'feeling words' tend to be nonspecific, often the catchall designations of "good," "bad," "sad," and "mad," rather than specific emotions like excited, surprised, delighted, relaxed, proud, hurt, scared, worried, bored, impatient, etc. When experiences are left unattended and unworded (let alone deliberately ignored or mislabeled), the acquisition and use of body-state and emotive language can be impacted. If your hunger is not named or attended to, if your discomfort is left unexplained, if your fatigue is not acknowledged, how would you know what to call the gurgles in your tummy, the burning of a rash, or the fuzzy droopy feeling of exhaustion, the pain of abuse?

Babies and young children have no way to attend to their own discomfort. When caregivers do not alleviate their suffering (even more so when caregivers cause it!), children's only means for relief is to escape their bodies by dissociating. Even if others talk about hunger, pain, joy, boredom, or sadness, children who are shut down cannot associate these words with internal experience. The words may remain meaningless unless children can relate them to how they are feeling. This disconnect does not automatically resolve if the child is removed from an overwhelming situation (Gaensbauer 2011). Because maltreated children may not know how to utilize offered care or how to ask for it, caregivers can find it difficult to decipher and respond to the child's messages. When their care fails to address the child's needs, it can inadvertently reinforce children's disconnection and comprehension of body states and emotive language.

Some foster or adoptive caregivers can be given conflicting recommendations about how to best support a child. They could be advised to let the child lead the way and remain attentive to cues for what the child needs, but when that child does not give cues they can interpret or does not respond as they expect, caregivers can be at a loss. The child might not cry or say that he/she is hungry; not be comforted by soothing; never seem satiated or ready to sleep. Other caregivers are advised to keep strict routines (e.g. similar to the one at the orphanage) for predictability, but the rigidity might disregard the child's individual needs and mask the child's real hunger and fatigue. Between the child's dissociation and the caregivers' possible misinterpretation of the child's emotions and needs, connection and communication can remain compromised.

Children whose pain or distress was not acknowledged or attended to might learn to ignore their bodies and may dissociate from sensations, emotions, and discomfort. Words about personal experience can feel foreign and confounding to them. Some children are afraid to have any needs, especially if those brought on confusion and pain or if to be cared for came with strings attached. Maltreated children often hide or deny sadness, pain, hunger, fatigue, anger. To recognize and identify needs and feelings can feel triggering. To feel may make real what was too painful to manage. This disconnection can also be true for children who experienced medical trauma (e.g. accidents, congenital issues, chronic pain). Children whose pain is undertreated, played down, or ignored can perceive themselves as somehow 'wrong' for having pain. They can become confused about what pain is or how real theirs is, especially if they are told that "this doesn't really hurt that much" or that "everything's okay" when things are not (Carter 2002, Kuttner 2010). Children may be too young or ill to inquire about relief or believe that to show pain or anger will lead to more hurting (e.g. if they believe that they are held down as punishment). Children may feel bad for the upset 'they' (i.e. their pain) bring up in their parent, may not cry or ask or try to explain, managing by dissociation instead.

Medical issues themselves often require ignoring body states. Hunger may not be sated (e.g. before procedures), or children may be fed when they are not hungry or in spite of feeling nauseated (e.g. upper GI tests). Body functions may no longer be under their control: "Needing to make" may have little meaning when there's incontinence, constant urgency from an infection or catheter, or an inability to call for a bedpan. Words like "no" and "stop" can be confusing, as can "good for you" and "worse" and "better" (e.g. "this will make you feel better" for something that does not for the child at that time). Medically ill children can have difficulty naming body states or emotions if they are numb and the words feel empty or do not matter.

Being dissociated from one's own body and feelings can make it difficult to recognize and label those in others too (Gaensbauer 2002, 2011, Fogassi & Ferrarri 2007, Ninio & Snow 1996, van der Kolk 2014). Traumatized children can seem to lack empathy or have odd interpretations for social situations. How children use words is always informative and offers a window to their interpretation of the world and their experience. A child may see an injured or crying person and say "happy" because she was told "aren't you happy the doctors came so fast?", but for her the arrival of the doctor is tied to pain and injury and it made her cry or feel like crying. She may just be guessing, arbitrarily applying a feeling word to a depiction of an emotional situation. The same child may also use "happy" in response to a birthday party or a present, reflecting the confusing experiences and meanings she might have inferred. A child who associates a sweaty person with maltreatment may not realize that someone wiping his or her face after a run is 'hot,' 'thirsty,' or 'sweaty.' Instead they may feel alarmed and say the person is 'mean.' If others respond with puzzled looks or laugh at the error, the child may feel ashamed, confused, even frightened.

All children make sense of their reality through the mirroring of adults (Cozolino 2006, 2014, Gaensbauer 2011, Halla 1999). If caregivers' words and actions match children's feeling and need, they learn to trust their perceptions and body sensations. They know to look to the adult for clues for differentiating and interpreting comfort and discomfort, pleasure and pain, worry and calm. An adult's interpretation often takes precedence over that of the child: If an adult is happy, it must mean that something good has happened; if the adult is angry, the child may believe she is bad or must have done something wrong. She may feel anxious and guilty whether she did or did not do anything wrong, believing she deserved it if anything bad does occur.

Sensitive adults validate the child's feelings even when these differ from their own. They will acknowledge the child's unhappiness for needing to stay with the babysitter as just as real as their own joy over going out on an anniversary date. This helps the child learn that there can be more than one feeling—and view—about a situation. However, if the adult does not notice (or care about) the child's emotion, the child may remain confused: Is her feeling awful a happy thing or a bad thing? Does happy mean feeling not good inside? Does happy mean someone else has to be sad?

Children who find body-state and emotive words confusing are less likely to use them. Maltreated children often use "I don't know" when asked about feelings, especially if feelings are something the child has little experience with identifying.

"The Meaning of Hope"—When Assumptions Derail Communication

The fourth graders brought their class assignment to the session, an essay about: "What I hope the world will be like when I am grown." All three boys in the inner-city public school had language-learning issues. They needed to comprehend the words before they could form a narrative response. I explained what 'grown' meant, then I asked them what 'hope' was and got blank faces. A discussion followed:

"Is hope a good thing or a bad thing?"(More blank faces) "Well," I prompted, undeterred. "If I say, 'I hope it will be nice outside tomorrow,' what do you think I mean?" (Silence) "Let's think together. Is hope something that makes people feel good, or feel bad?" The kids gazed around the room as if the walls had suddenly sprouted fascinating vistas, then a brave soul took a chance, "Um . . . Miss Y, maybe a bad thing?"

"A bad thing? Okay, how come?"

"I don't know"—shrug. "I just thinking it a bad feeling thing . . . "

There was a pregnant pause, then another child chimed in, "Yeah, it bad because it is like, everything is only being mess up already, so when I grow up it will be more mess up . . . "

Nods galore.

This went beyond comprehension delay and missing concepts—it was their reality communicated. The boys (and too many other children who have hope-deprived upbringings) had very little experience with hope that wasn't drowned by disappointment and failed promises. They were given little to hope for and were constantly flagged for their failures, not their successes. Many saw them as failing kids in a failing school in a failing neighborhood of failing families. Their life experiences (and possibly those of their parents) gave them little reason to imagine things bettered. No wonder they found it difficult to conceive of "hope" as anything but something disheartening.

How do you define "hope" to someone who does not know it? Yet it is never more important than for those whose situations may seem hopeless. So I began with something the boys understood: a drawing competition where they could "hope to win" a small reward. We called that flutter of excitement they felt "hope" (they all 'won' for some 'artistic skill'). We hoped for good weather so they would get to play outside for recess, and the next session we hoped that the microwave-cookies we were improvising would come out edible (they did not, and we all laughed as I resorted to store-bought backup). We discussed how hope does not mean we will get what we had hoped for but can still make us feel good inside. We hoped all kinds of things: a win for the baseball team, pizza and not mystery meat at lunch. And a seed for the concept was planted, even as we also discussed pride, satisfaction, joy, excitement, calm . . .

A couple of weeks later I asked the boys nonchalantly what 'hope' meant. They rolled eyes at me and one responded: "Something you feel good when you thinking about it because you wait and maybe it happens and you be real happy." Another boy, a bit starry eyed, added: "I hope one day that I not live in the projects no more and we have no more roaches and that my brother he not live with my first dad anymore but he come live with me."

My students taught me that hope is not something to take for granted: It needs to be allowed, cultivated, and learned. Words like happy, confident, proud, successful, peaceful, and content must also be connected to reality like umbilical cords to fetuses—they should be nourished before they can breathe independently.

(A version of this excerpt first appeared as "Teaching Hope" in *ISSTD* [International Society for the Study of Trauma and Dissociation] *News* 2007)

Cause-and-Effect

Children learn cause and its effect through opportunities to explore what happens when they do things. Well-cared-for babies learn early that caregivers make things better. When they quiet at the sound of their parent's footsteps or voice, they show us they have learned to anticipate relief when their caregiver approaches and have learned it from all the times when relief followed the caregiver's presence, footsteps, or voice. Predictions become more complex as infants grow: Calling out brings people; letting go of the bottle makes it fall; smiling makes others smile back; throwing food on the floor brings the dog. They learn that if they move a certain way they can reach things; that touching some things will bring on a firm "no!" Normally developing well-cared-for babies constantly test their hypotheses, in part to confirm their understanding of causation and in part to exercise their growing sense of control over their world. Infants will deliberately reach over to touch a forbidden item and pause to anticipate the caregiver's "no." They may repeat it, delighted that it 'works.' Repetition teaches babies what to expect as well as the boundaries of what is allowed and the impact of their actions, vocalizations, smiles, and cries (Baron 1992, de Boysson-Bardies 1999, Cozolino 2006, Ninio & Snow 1996, Schore 2012, Siegel 2012). Predictability reassures and confirms. It is why young children ask for the same stories, songs, and videos and laugh at 'knock-knock' jokes.

To understand cause-and-effect requires the child be aware of what is happening around him and have opportunities to experiment with things and reactions. Children who have insufficient opportunities for exploring and relational exchanges have less mastery over their environment, and their ability to predict may be compromised. They might not understand how one thing leads to another, how or what might happen and why. These difficulties can be especially marked in institutionalized and/or severely neglected children following parental inability, mental illness, addiction, and overwhelm (Albers et al 2005, De Bellis 2005, Miller 2005). The children may spend hours in cribs with limited access to toys, activity, and other people. They could be fed or changed when adults remember rather than in response to their hunger or discomfort.

Sounds and actions may become associated (e.g. the light going on with caregivers' approach), but children may have little opportunity to affect these actions. Crying may not bring people to comfort them. Vocalizing may not bring smiles. Hunger may not mean they will be fed. Things happen around them and to them but are not in reaction to their voice, need, or antics.

Neglected babies may show limited interest in initiating play or experimentation. Even when provided with toys, they may not know what to do with them (Albers et al 2005, Miller 2005, Silberg 1998). They may not look to see where a bottle fell because an adult wasn't there to look down, pick up the bottle, and narrate what happened. They may not realize that they can cause an effect. They may not know that crying can be used to call someone. They may not know that people's presence can bring relief.

Abused children often have more opportunities to experiment than severely neglected children do, but if their attempts were met with anger or resulted in frightening responses, their curiosity might be curtailed. If smiling can just as easily elicit a smile or a slap and "what are you smiling at?", babies may be less likely to connect smiling with pleasant interaction or reciprocation (Vissing et al 1991). Medically traumatized children may also fear exploration. If touching things brought pain, they may be afraid to try to do things. They could try not to move much if they are already hurt. Unable to predict what may or may not bring on pain, traumatized children may limit their vocalization and crying, activity, social gestures, and variation on play (Casey et al 1996, Danon-Boileau 2002, Doesburg et al 2013, Ford & Courtois 2013, Gaensbauer 2002, Heineman 1998, Heller & Lapierre 2012, Kuttner 2010, Pearce & Pezzot-Pearce 1997, Silberg 1998).

Helplessness is a devastating feeling. Traumatized children try to find some control by believing they are somehow to blame (Gomez 2012, Silberg 2013, Wieland 2011). Such misconceptions are often reinforced by adults who say: "Why did you do that?! Look what you've done! It's your fault for crying/making noise/messing your diaper/spilling milk/dropping your bottle ..."

Trapped between needing to affect change (i.e. get help, be fed, feel loved) and fearing it, they get overwhelmed. Hypervigilant children may not know which of many stimuli had caused the reaction, while numb children may be unable to understand the cause-and-effect of things they were not sufficiently present for. An already scary world can become even more disjointed when the child does not know what to expect or what may happen.

Sequence

Sequence includes the understanding that things happen in a certain order: Socks go on first, then shoes; you are uncomfortable → you cry → someone comes → wet diaper is removed → you are clean and dry → you feel better. Babies learn sequence through routines that follow certain patterns and through the narratives and explanations that reinforce them. A caregiver says: "Oh, I know, you are hungry. Let me make a bottle for you. I'll put some milk in the bottle and warm it up for you. Give me one more minute, Sweetie, it is almost ready. Yes, I know it's hard to wait. All ready, there you go, nice and yummy?" The baby becomes familiar with the steps that eventually bring the bottle, and as soon as she sees the caregiver take an empty bottle, she knows it will be filled, then warmed, then given to her. She knows that the discomfort in her belly will be followed by food and satiety.

When events happen haphazardly, babies may find it difficult to learn what to expect next: Sometimes things take place, sometimes they do not; food may or may not appear; it may or may not get to the baby's mouth. It may bring pain and not relief (too hot, too cold, spoiled, colic, not being burped). A caregiver may pick the baby up to feed her or walk right past and not return for what feels like an eternity. There is no sequence for events. Things can start and never end. The same cue can lead to comfort or overwhelm.

Maltreated children often struggle with sequence and temporal order (what needs to happen first, second, etc.) (Nadeau & Nolin 2013, Pearce & Pezzot-Pearce 1997, Putnam 1997, Yehuda 2005, 2011). Chaos and unpredictability combine with overwhelm and dissociation to render the world capricious. Reality may already be incomprehensible: One minute you are playing quietly in your room and the next you are slapped without knowing why; you go to school not knowing who you will go home to; you don't know if you will be fed. When children dissociate to manage overwhelm, their awareness of what is taking place becomes limited. They can end up with fragmented understanding because they missed parts of what happened, reinforcing feelings of unpredictability.

If sequence and order are too vague, children can find it hard to understand how events unfolded in a story, what needs to happen first or next. They may list people or actions but not know why things happen one way and not another. Pictures of a story may seem unrelated rather than depicting a connected narrative. Explanations may be disjointed, reflecting the idiosyncrasies of their world's unpredictability.

For some children, having to arrange a sequence can be scary. For them to be asked "what should you do now?" or "what happened next?" can elicit confusion from times things happened they could not explain. They may realize that they are not 'getting' something that they should, and fear reprisal if they had been punished for not knowing things. Putting things in order can trigger memories of pain if abusive caregivers accompanied abuse with: "You know what's coming now . . .", "What did you think would happen?" Children may also have good reason to not internalize sequence if how one thing led to another was overwhelming. Better to not make connections between what takes place now and what it says about what is about to happen (e.g. "Mom is drinking → she gets mean → hits you" or "bedtime arrived → you go to sleep → Dad comes into bedroom → does bad things"). It could feel safer to not connect the dots, not have to think about it, not have to know.

Narrative

Narrative provides the story of one's experiences, actions, motivations, thoughts, and perceptions. It describes people, places, events, feelings, ideas, and impressions. It allows the verbal depiction of aspirations, plans, and recollections. It reflects understanding of concepts and one's views of others and the world. Narrative can offer a measure of communication abilities because it relies on comprehension and the ability to access vocabulary for expression, is shaped by the understanding of how things work, and takes the knowledge of the listener into account by providing sufficient details to give a sense of what took place (Berman 2004, Gleason & Ratner 2009, Ninio & Snow 1996).

Children learn narrative from their caregivers (Baron 1992, Berman 2004, de Boysson-Bardies 1999). Every time caregivers talk to babies about where they are going and what they'll see or do, each time caregivers verbalize for infants what they may be experiencing and feeling, when caregivers recount what babies did or read a bedtime story—babies are exposed to narrative and learn how it can be used to weave events and experiences with words. Narrative is a complex skill that develops throughout childhood and often throughout life. However, all of its aspects are present in simplified but effective forms by preschool age (Berman 2004, Gleason & Ratner 2009, Heymann 2010). Even young children can tell stories about where they went, who they saw, what they want to be when they grow up, what happened in the movies when their popcorn spilled or at the doctor's when their baby brother got a shot.

Given how vocabulary, body state, emotive language, cause-effect, and sequence can be impacted by trauma, it should not be surprising that narrative abilities in traumatized children often suffer as well (Pearce & Pezzot-Pearce 1997, Putnam 1997, Silberg 1998, Yehuda 2005). Children who have fragmented perception of reality and experiences can struggle to put together cohesive narrative. Children who are not used to being listened to (and/or feeling heard) and have had few narratives that were relevant to their needs may have fewer 'building blocks' for making stories. Their narratives can come across as skeletal, literal, or ambiguous and hard to follow. In addition, the very stories traumatized children try to tell are of events that were fragmented and confusing, which makes them harder to construct and comprehend. Gaps in children's stories can mirror and reflect the gaps in their awareness and the disjointed experience of overwhelm they live.

Literal, Ambiguous, and Symbolic Meaning

Ambiguity, metaphor, and symbolism are part of language. Words can have more than one meaning (e.g. "Duck!"), and sentences can mean different things depending on how and where they are said (e.g. "Is the window open?" by someone shivering in winter or sweaty in summer). Symbolic language phrases can mean something very different than their words (e.g. "I'm all ears"), and metaphors depict things that do not quite make sense (e.g. "the sun danced on the water"). Multiple meanings and symbolism enrich our communication and add layers of context and innuendo to narrative and discourse. They can also be quite confusing to young children.

Children learn to listen to what people say, so when words don't match what they think they heard, it can throw them off. Young children are literal. Why did Mommy say she "had something in the back of her head all day"—there is nothing there! What does it mean that someone "eats like a bird?" Do they eat worms? It takes exposure, time, and maturation for a child to entertain two meanings simultaneously and to understand expressions and metaphors. Rich language, literacy, legends, stories, and conversation expose children to puns and idioms in context and help them realize that when words don't match, there is a 'hidden' meaning to infer (Berman 2004, Brinton & Fujiki 1989, Gleason & Ratner 2009, Heymann 2010, Ninio & Snow 1996).

Processing ambiguity and symbolic language requires listening, attention, processing, curiosity, and flexibility—all things that are difficult to do when overwhelmed (Siegel 2012, van der Kolk 2014). Traumatized children often miss nuances in stories and narrative. To understand symbolic language, children need to listen to the literal meaning of the words in context while simultaneously holding an alternate hypothesis about the words meaning something different. They need to maintain attention to process the context in which the expression was heard to know which one fits. This level of processing is difficult to do when one is overwhelmed, hypervigilant, or shut down. Traumatized children often find symbolic language confusing, and the confusion can add stress and reinforce dissociation, causing the child to miss even more. In addition, the ambiguous and 'tricky-sounding' language can remind a traumatized child of times when adults said things they could not understand and yet were somehow expected to. It can trigger anxiety over what is going on and what it could mean. Children may believe that they are being tricked on purpose or lied to. They may get angry and aggressive, unable to explain what triggered them to feel unsafe, scared, or shut down. Semantics weave the world around us into meaning. When language fails to do so, it loses some of its connective tissue and becomes less relationally rewarding. It can affect how we use language, what we use it for, and how well we can rely on it for communicating our reality.

10 Trauma's Impact on Pragmatics

Language Use, Social Cues, and Discourse Rules

Pragmatics refers to the ways we use communication—the communicative intent of the interaction: questioning, answering, noting, inquiring, commenting, ordering, confirming, denying, clarifying, etc. It includes the roles one has in an interaction (e.g. speaker, listener, teacher, narrator) and the rules by which we interact: take turns, wait our turn, keep to a topic, change a topic and respond to such a shift, take the listener's knowledge into account, use and understand humor and sarcasm, offer new information, and manage miscommunications. By definition, pragmatics requires a communication partner. It is learned, evolving from basic reciprocity of gazing, smiling, and turn-taking in peek-a-boo and cooing in babies to the complex social understanding of what topics one may bring up in what way in what company, or which euphemism one might use and why (Baron 1992, Berman 2004, de Boysson-Bardies 1999, Gleason & Ratner 2009, Halla 1999, Ninio & Snow 1996).

Every language in the world includes pragmatic rules. Some communication intents such as seeking information, requesting, denying, and greeting are universal, though the ways they are used may vary by culture. In some cultures, children may not be encouraged to ask questions, denial is oblique, direct inquiry or display of unpleasant emotions is considered impolite. Interaction rules and polite language such as 'thank you' and 'excuse me'; greetings like 'hello' and 'how do you do'; and gestures used for accepting, parting, and negating are also often culture dependent, context dependent, and speaker dependent. We greet our boss differently than our child, interact differently in a football game and a funeral, may use formal versus familiar language, and must know where, when, and how to respond to social settings.

Pragmatics is a crucial aspect of language competency. It provides the substrate for understanding context, meaning, and intent. Gaffes in communication are often errors in pragmatic application. Pragmatic errors by people learning a new language in a new culture make them stand out as 'different' or 'newcomers,' at least as much as pronunciation or semantic errors do. Children make pragmatic errors, too—raise their voices at the library, ask direct questions about delicate topics, share too-personal information, misjudge a change of topic, etc. Such errors from young children are usually met with chuckles, an indulging smile, and gentle correction. The same errors are less mildly tolerated from older children, because pragmatics includes social expectations about the behavior of persons of various ages and standing (Bell et al 1986, Brinton & Fujiki 1989, Halla 1999, Ninio & Snow 1996). Clumsy pragmatics often gets people feeling uncomfortable around persons with developmental disabilities, autism, or the mentally ill. A person's vocabulary and grammar can be acceptable or superior, but if their pragmatics is 'off' they may be judged as obtuse, impolite, or socially inept.

Pragmatic skills are learned through exposure and rehearsal. Children observe and internalize the rules and customs of their environment from interactions others have with them and from what they see when others interact. Everyday exchanges teach children about questions and replies, noting and commenting, greeting, turn-taking, requesting, and more. Well-cared-for children utilize some pragmatic skill even before words appear, with the variety and complexity of pragmatics evolving throughout childhood (Berman 2004, Gleason & Ratner 2009, Ninio & Snow 1996).

Maltreatment and Pragmatics

Maltreatment and overwhelm can impact children's comprehension of pragmatics and their repertoire of communicative intents. They might only use a limited repertoire of communication intents, and the 'rules' they infer from their reality (e.g. respond but not initiate, do not inquire) may not match those of society (Pearce & Pezzot-Pearce 1997, Silberg 2013, Yehuda 2005). Neglected children may not know how to apply social rules if they haven't had enough exposure and practice, and abused children may find some interactions frightening (e.g. if asking for something or initiating meant being hurt).

The relationships children are exposed to affect their pragmatics, as do presence of mind and awareness. A shut-down child cannot attend to social cues and will miss communication, and a hypervigilant child may be too activated to 'read' social possibilities in an interaction (Putnam 1997, Silberg 1998, Wieland 2011, Yehuda 2011). Overwhelm curtails curiosity and listening. It affects relatedness, awareness, and attunement, all of which are paramount to pragmatic communication (Cozolino 2014, van der Kolk 2014). Traumatized children can appear to be—and can feel—like 'outsiders' in interactions, and their issues and social awkwardness place them at high risk for bullying or being bullied (Eliot & Cornell 2009, Espelage et al 2000, Takizawa et al 2014). The rules they learned might be that it is acceptable to take your anger out on others and torment the weak, that humiliating others is funny or depicts power. They can misinterpret jokes as insults and 'punish' others for disagreeing or showing different opinions than theirs. Even traumatized children who do not fall into the bully/

bullied dynamic can become or feel like outsiders. They may be too occupied with managing pain, hurt, worry, anxiety, and triggers to engage socially (Drew 2007, Kuttner 2010), may not know how to appropriately show interest in others, and may find others who are interested in them scary or intrusive (Vissing et al 1991, Rogers & Williams 2006).

Normally developing children are intensely social. They discuss things they saw or heard, things they played with, where they went, or what they want to do. They exchange fantasies and concoct whole scenarios for play, moving fluidly in and out of roles and communicative intents. They adore jokes and silliness. Not so for maltreated children, for whom interactions can feel foreign, confusing, and even frightening, who may not be able to (or be allowed to) talk about their lives, and may not understand how other children can. Children can feel ashamed of the realities they live—a foster-home, a parent in jail—and believe they are at fault (Bennett et al 2010). They may worry that others will laugh at or not believe them. Some try to bluff their way to fitting in by making up stories, only to overreact and interpret any questions as challenges, leading to negative responses from others (Yehuda 2011). Children can push friendly peers, yearning for connection but not knowing how to 'be social' (Lyons-Ruth et al 2009, Silberg 2013, Wieland 2011).

Medical Trauma and Pragmatics

In some children, trauma may only temporarily disrupt overall good care (e.g. medical trauma, natural disaster, war). However, even children who have good pragmatics may struggle with social cues when they are activated and may become confused when social rules change during crisis. Children may believe that refusal is no longer allowed or that only adults are allowed to ask questions (Carter 2002, Kuttner 2010, Shiminski-Maher 1993). Sick children may find it hard to connect with peers who do not understand (and may be disgusted by) their world of treatments, chemo, hair loss, weakness, and possible dying. Older children may want to fit in but be out of the loop. The medical reality itself, along with pain, medications, and treatment side effects can also impact pragmatics: Children may feel detached, numb, tired, and less able to engage. They may find social discourse hard to follow, miss punch lines and parts of conversations. They may become hypersensitive to perceived rejection and intolerant of misunderstandings, pushing friends away, yet feeling devastated when those friends pull back (Drew 2007).

Social interactions can be difficult for ill or visibly disabled children, yet even more so for maltreated children, whose struggle is almost always invisible. A child whose behavior is unpleasant or who becomes 'no longer fun to be with' may see peers (and often adults) staying away. Rejection makes further interactions stressful and increases likelihood for more gaffes. While adults often try to stay engaged with a distressed child, even they might keep their distance if a child is constantly prickly. Children, who are naturally egocentric, may just look to someone else to play with. Both directly and indirectly, trauma can impact children's pragmatics and socialization. The following sections detail various pragmatic aspects and how they might manifest in children with developmental trauma.

Turn-Taking and Reciprocity—Responding, Initiating, and Following and Giving Directions

Benjamin was nine months old and had recently discovered crawling and pulling himself to a stand. His father, his main caregiver, worked from home and was sitting on the couch with the laptop. The baby played quietly a while but was bored and looking for engagement. Benjamin crawled to his dad's foot, climbed up, and held on to the man's pant leg, grinning in delight. Benjamin's dad continued to stare at the screen, making no eye contact. The baby babbled but the father still did not respond. Benjamin screeched and bounced up and down. The movement shifted the computer and Benjamin's father lifted it, frowned at the baby, and pried the little hands off of his pants. "Stop it!" he said. "Get off." He turned the baby away and plopped him on the floor an arm's length away. Benjamin sat quietly for a second, then twisted to gaze at his father but the adult ignored him. When Benjamin tried to stand again, the father moved his leg and Benjamin fell on his bottom. His face crumbled and he cried, but his father did not respond. After a while, Benjamin quieted, curled up away from his father, and fell asleep. When Benjamin's mother returned home in the evening, the baby was clingy, and cried whenever she tried to put him down. "Let him cry," the father stated. "You are spoiling him. He doesn't give me any trouble because he knows I won't have any of this clinginess."

§

Manuel was thirteen months old. He spent the first eleven months of his life in an orphanage after being abandoned as a newborn, and his adoptive mother was worried. The boy did not turn when she called his name, made no eye contact, and rarely babbled. He rocked a lot. The pediatrician suspected he may be deaf, but a hearing test showed normal otoacoustic emissions and a brisk auditory reflex. Manuel's mother was not surprised: She believed he could hear but was uninterested in human sounds. Her worry was autism. Manuel had been in a room with many infants of varied ages. The few caregivers kept the babies fed and clean, but interaction and personal contact were limited. Infants did not leave their cribs much or have opportunities for play because toys were kept out of cribs for safety reasons.

Though healthy, Manuel was only in the 10th percentile for head circumference and his motor skills were underdeveloped. "I don't think he knows what to do with people," his adoptive mother worried. "He seems so lost."

Interaction is an innate need, and everyday routines usually provide infants with a plethora of communication opportunities. Maltreated babies also seek contact, but the rules they learn may be different than those that well-cared-for babies do. The unkind response of Benjamin's father was not outright abusive, but if their exchange was representative of his ongoing care, Benjamin could learn that initiating is not welcome. On his end, the baby tried all his communication skills: He sought proximity, vocalized, tried to attract attention via social gesture and smiling; even reattempted contact after his father refused it. What got communicated back was that his interaction was unwanted and he will not be attended to. Benjamin's brief crying and how he curled up to sleep away from his father may be telling us he learned to shut down and wait for his mommy to come home. His clinginess to her may reflect his attempts to communicate his anger and confusion. She may provide opportunities for reparative interaction, but his desperate clinging to his tired mother who has only limited time with him puts Benjamin at risk for not acquiring a full range of pragmatic interaction and communication.

Neglect stunts pragmatic growth. Like Manuel, babies from communicatively deprived environments may not know how to reciprocate and interact. They may cry little, stop babbling, not realize that eye contact is how one can engage, or know to respond to their names. Some may find environmental sounds more interesting than human ones (Albers et al 2005, De Bellis 2005, Miller 2005). Abused babies may shy away from communication because reciprocity meant fear and harm (Vissing et al 1991). Babies learn to look away, shut down, and not respond. They may seek comfort in objects, not people. Such behaviors often lead to misdiagnoses of autism, even though they do not reflect an inability to communicate. They may actually be quite effective communicators of their reality, and the intervention they need is often very different than for autism.

Manuel indeed had difficulties with the basic rules of social interaction and communication—but he was neither deaf nor autistic. His turning away was not rejection of his adoptive parents' care but a reflection of what he had known. To help him, Manuel's adoptive parents went back to basics (see Chapter 15) and learned how to offer regulation and simple dyadic interaction, reinforce occasional eye contact, and encourage vocalizations. Their care built pathways that his early life had disrupted. Tentatively and then more frequently, Manuel began reciprocating. He made eye contact, responded, vocalized. He learned to protest and deny as well as to accept and welcome; he greeted, smiled, and began vocalizing in response. He took turns and learned to interact and talk.

When Listening to 'How' Meant a Lot More Than What Was Said

During communication one needs to understand what is said and simultaneously infer intent from the context and the interaction. Well-cared-for normally developing children show an amazing ability for this dual processing. Kindergarteners can respond to "is the window open?" with 'yes' or 'no' while also understanding that the question was a request for action: have the window opened or closed depending on how hot or cold the person is. They can comprehend semantics and pragmatics simultaneously: the question as well as why it was asked. This processing can be difficult for traumatized children, and their assumptions about intention may not fit the current context.

Stella, age eight, was in special education and struggled with comprehension and completing assignments. Born to an addicted mother, Stella was often left for hours in the crib while the mother looked for a 'fix' or was in a stupor from one. She was almost three when Child Protective Services removed her to 'family foster-care,' where she bounced between relatives before being transferred to a stable foster-home. The girl was quiet but withdrawn. It was easy to forget she was even in class. She did not fight, fidget, protest, or make noise. She made what seemed like very careless mistakes, like omitting important steps or failing to apply things she had just been taught. It drove the teacher and the foster-mother nuts. "I just showed you how to do this!" they would sputter, raising their hands in dismay at whatever got done completely wrong. "You did the total opposite! Why didn't you tell me if you didn't understand?"

It was likely that Stella had neurological damage from exposure to substances in the womb. She also suffered a difficult and lonely beginning, suffered discomfort, need, and many disruptions. She learned to shut down, place few demands, and attend to people's mood rather than their words. Her mother would get irritable and scary, and Stella coped by learning to be quiet and asking for nothing. Her biological mother's rambling and cursing rarely made sense. Only her tone did. When Stella's foster-parent—a kind but boomingly demonstrative woman—raised her voice to explain, Stella could not listen. She was focused on the woman's face and body language, anticipating pain. It would happen in school, too. Overfocusing on 'how' people communicated left Stella little space for listening to what they actually said.

When Intent Is Intolerable—When Comprehension Means Pain

How we interact with children forms their sense of themselves and their place in the world (Cozolino 2006, 2014, Schore 2012, Siegel 2012, van der Kolk 2014). Our words as well as the intent we communicate become a child's reality. Sensitive caregivers communicate children's value to them by the care they provide as well as the opportunities they allow for the child's intent to be communicated and how they respond to what a child wants but is not possible. Children learn that their caregivers' decisions come from care, and empathetic responses to unacceptable choices communicate to children that their input matters even if they cannot have their way (Landry et al 2006a, Ninio & Snow 1996, Stams et al 2002).

The situation is different for children who are maltreated by their caregivers. The helplessness of childhood is magnified when those who are supposed to keep you safe are sources of danger, pain, and overwhelm. Children are locked into impossible double-binds: The very ones they depend on for safety are those who violate it (Giovanni 2004, Liotti 2009, Lyons-Ruth & Block 1996, Lyons-Ruth et al 2006). To comprehend that your caregiver intends to harm you is intolerable; to accept that the person you need for existence wishes you never existed is intolerable. Children are unable to change this intentional reality but can change their awareness of it: They dissociate, disengage, minimize, forget, ignore, deny.

"A Mistake"—Gabby: Necessary Denial

Ten-year-old Gabby was a mistake. Her mother never intended for her to be born. She "made her kids early" and "got them out of the house." She did not want "another drooling pooper to wipe after." Everything about Gabby made her mother angry and she couldn't stand the baby's constant need. Gabby grew up on a daily diet of "you're a mistake," "I never wanted you," "my life was finally perfect before you showed up and ruined it," "you are ugly," "I should have aborted you when I had the chance," and other soul-crushing assaults. She learned to walk on eggshells, ask for nothing, and anticipate everything her mom might need. She learned to not make noises when she ate because those reminded her mom that she was "eating up her money." She learned to hide being sick so that her mother would not get angry she "got sick to get attention." Gabby accepted that every-thing was—had to be—her fault; that if she were somehow better, faster, quieter, cleaner, more caring, more sensitive, more something, her mother would find some room in her heart to love her. It had to be only because of her unacceptable flaws and ugliness of her being that her mother did not love her. She had to be so awful. How could her mother love her?

In spite of everything (for the alternative was to be crushed by sorrow), Gabby idolized her mother. She made up stories about the things they did together. She found excuses for missing permission slips for field trips her mother refused to sign (because Gabby "did not deserve it"), for her mother never coming to parent-teacher conferences, for the books that were not bought and Gabby said she had lost. She manufactured an alternative reality, and when people caught her in a lie and pun-ished her for it, she accepted it just as she took the blame when teachers scolded her for "losing" the permission slip or not bringing money for picture day. Gabby already believed she was at fault, anyway, for everything. It was also easier to be blamed than to have others know—and be confronted with the reality—that her mother did not love her enough to care.

Gabby could not afford to let in her mother's communications, so she constructed her own interpretation of what her mother had to mean: If she was only good enough, she would be loved; if she did not ask or demand, she might be accepted; if others thought her mother loved her, it may become truth. She reinterpreted communication to make reality marginally tolerable. Like Gabby, maltreated children can be both desperate for and suspicious of praise, and can interpret the mildest critique as proof of blame. They may not know how to argue or negotiate, may not ask for clarification, they may not initiate if they do not know how or believe they haven't the right to be curious.

Inquiry and Curiosity

While it is not limited to childhood (or humans), curiosity is a hallmark of the young as they play, explore, flail, fall flat, and try again. Playfulness allows practice of later-needed skills and builds resilience for later challenges through the small conflicts and stressors of play such as chasing and catching (Konner 2010). Interpersonal inquiry and curiosity often involve language, and as anyone who spent time with a three-year-old knows, children can become quite masterful at queries (Berman 2004, Ninio & Snow 1996). This endearing (if at times exasperating) behavior cannot take place if a child is not allowed to ask, is scared to, or if curiosity proved painful. It cannot happen if a child is overwhelmed. A dissociated child cannot be curious. Hypervigilant children are reactive and alert to danger, not exploration: They may ask repetitively for reassurance, not learning (Silberg 1998, 2013, Wieland 2011, Yehuda 2011).

Trauma, illness, and stress squelch curiosity and exploration by contracting energy around survival. Orphaned elephant and rhino calves will not play, feed, and interact and can literally die of grief (Newberry & Swanson 2008). When sick or stressed children play, their play is often muted (Kuttner 2010) or lacks imagination (Silberg 1998). Chronically traumatized children may not know how to be curious even when opportunities arise. School may offer many interesting things, but if a child does not know how to engage with them or respond to them, they will fall behind. Curiosity can be scary if it brought on pain, and the excitement of something new can be tamped down by anxiety. Maltreated children may not know they are allowed to get up and get something, touch things, or ask about what they do not understand. They can come across as passive and disinterested when they are actually numb and unaware that curiosity is allowed to them. They may be aggressive and stereotypical, not knowing how to explore (Levine & Kline 2007, Osofsky 2011, Pearce & Pezzot-Pearce 1997, Silberg 1998, Yehuda 2005).

If 'No' Did Not Matter and Neither Did 'Please'

Social language includes polite engagement through "please, "thank you," "sorry," and "have a good day," as well as social gestures like body movements and facial expressions (Ninio & Snow 1996). Culturally mediated rules of hierarchy and authority dictate who can say what to whom, when, and in what way. They define what is expected of a person of a certain age (or gender, or status) and how one behaves in different company. Like all pragmatics, social language is fluid, with rules that can shift over time and place. Children are expected to speak to their parents in a different way than they speak to their siblings, grandparents, or a stranger. They learn an 'inside voice' for class, library, or store and where to use a more rambunctious 'outside voice.' We teach social language when we remind children to use the "magic words" of please and thank you, or when we ask them to apologize for pushing someone or inadvertently messing up. Hopefully they see the same toward them: when they are thanked for handing over the bottle, when "please" is added to a request to clean up or to use less noise, when they are apologized to.

Teaching social language can go very differently for traumatized children, and their behavior may reflect it. Maltreated children can be rude because they were not shown how not to be. Some have learned how to apply rules in only very limited settings or with very few people and do not have pragmatic flexibility (Briscoe-Smith & Hinshaw 2006, Cohen 2001, Cole et al 2005, Eliot & Cornell 2009, Gaensbauer 2011, Silberg 2013, Yehuda 2005, 2011). They can appear clumsy, loud, too shy, or too boisterous. They may not know to wait their turn or to address a person appropriately. They may grab and push rather than ask. Paradoxically, they can also come across as polite to a fault, be wary of taking any chances, and 'adopt' others' opinions rather than voicing their own. They may apologize constantly even for things that are not their fault. They may refuse things they want because they do not believe they deserve them, or because they were punished when they did accept.

Social words need to be taught in context to make sense. If "please" had no connection to a genuine request, children may see "please" as designating an order and get upset when they do not get what they "asked for," or they may believe they must give something up if "please" was used and get aggressive in refusal. Some may not recognize a prompt like "how do you ask nicely?" (e.g. if they omit 'please') and not know what they did badly. For others, "asking nicely" may be a reminder of empty promises or awfulness.

Even deceptively simple "yes" and "no" can be confusing and not always about facts (e.g. is this a dog?). "Yes/no" can also communicate acceptance, approval, promising, denial, and refusal. If "yes" could not be trusted, children might grab what they can, ignore lack of permission, and take what they were refused. "No" may not mean much if it was all they heard or if theirs was unattended. They might sneak things and lie. Their history may have taught them that lying is something people do to get away with what they do not want to give back or deal with. Behavior is communication: When children's behavior changes or does not match social expectations, we need to take into account that they learned to engage through how others engaged with them and how they understood it.

"Please No!"—Doug: When Rules Fail

Five-year-old Doug was hurt in a car accident. His mother was still trapped in the driver's seat when the paramedics lifted him out of his and tied him onto a board. His leg was broken and he was bleeding from where glass shards embedded in his arm and face. He was in excruciating pain and feeling terrified. His mom was screaming but he could not see her, and the people did not take him to her. Instead, they took him away and kept hurting him. He cried "No!" when they stripped his clothes off and he screamed "Stop it!" but the strangers just continued making him naked and touched him everywhere—even where his mommy said no one should; especially when you said not to.

The people took him away from his mother. They didn't listen when he yelled for her. They just lied "it's okay" when it wasn't. None of it was okay. His parents told him not to go with strangers. They said if he was lost and alone, he should tell people to take him home, but these strangers tied him up and hurt him and took him away from his mommy. Even the police did not stop them. The police didn't listen when he needed help. His mommy always said the police would take him home if he got lost, but they didn't. They let the people take him somewhere different, away from his mommy. Everything was wrong.

One of the hurting people held his arm down. He had a needle. Doug was scared. Whenever he was due to have a shot at the doctor, his mommy told him in the morning beforehand, so he had time to get used to it, and she always held him afterward and he got to choose a treat. But his mommy wasn't there and no one told him about this shot and it hurt when the ambulance was moving and everything was scary and he had no clothes on. Everything was wrong. Doug even tried to ask pretty please to not do the shot, but the man just said, "Be still please. It's for your own good. So you'll feel better." This was not a real 'please'—the man didn't even wait for Doug to say okay—he just stuck him with the needle and it wasn't good for him and it didn't make him feel better. It only made his arm hurt more. Why did the man say 'please' if he didn't mean it? Why didn't the man listen when Doug cried "please no"?

All the things his mommy told him didn't work. Maybe magic words and safe rules and 'no' and 'stop' didn't matter anymore. Maybe he was really bad and he was being punished because he didn't say 'please' when he took a cookie and forgot his manners. Maybe it was his fault that the magic words and safe rules and promises were all broken.

Doug was a well-cared-for child, but the trauma of the car accident and what followed overwhelmed him and shattered his worldview for long after his physical wounds healed. His mother had been trapped and too badly hurt to be able to comfort him and it was a while before his father arrived from out of state to be with him. In the long hours Doug was alone, even though people checked on him constantly and no one was intentionally unkind, he experienced repeated disintegration of everything he knew about the world and how it was supposed to work. He was also delirious with pain and then drowsy and nauseated with pain medication, sensations he did not understand and which made everything harder to process and understand. The accident changed him. He no longer knew what to trust or whom. No promise felt real. He no longer believed that he had any power. He was terrified to be alone, yet was not comforted by his parents' presence—Doug no longer believed they could protect him or that their presence meant safety (more about Doug in Chapter 16).

When Questions Were Not Meant to Be Answered

Questions and answers form the basis of many exchanges: We seek and impart information, inquire and share, clarify and elaborate. We request new information ("Where were you Sunday night?"), seek confirmation about things we already know ("So, you will be there at five?"), ask rhetorically as a way to point out ("Did you see what just happened!?"), greet ("How are you?"), emote ("Can you believe this man!?"), request ("Is the window open?"), use sarcasm ("Anything else you think I should do before I can finally watch the game?"), wrap a command in politer form ("Would you step behind the white line, Ma'am?"), and more. Questions are the glue that holds together many conversations, and understanding the myriad ways questions can be utilized and their expected responses is part of pragmatic language use (Berman 2004, Brinton & Fujiki 1989, Halla 1999, Nippold 2007, Ninio & Snow 1996).

Until they acquire more sophisticated expressive skills, children tend to answer all questions—rhetorical or not—literally. However, even very young children grasp that questions carry communication intents that go beyond a verbal answer or gesture. If a preschooler is asked: "Did you see your brother's pacifier?" the child will answer yes or no but is likely to look around for the pacifier or add: "Daddy put it in the stroller." They understand both the question and the reason behind it as well as the expected response.

Maltreatment can result in a different understanding of questions. A child who heard questions framed as blaming commands ("What did you do?" "Why did you do it?" "What did I tell you about touching my stuff?") may not realize that a question is a query for information. They may get anxious at questions like: "What is your favorite ice cream flavor?", not knowing what they are expected to do or say. Children might mumble "I don't know" if they had no opportunities to develop preferences or might not dare voice opinions when they are not sure if those are the 'right ones.' Many had all decisions made for them, regardless of preference and without options for input. Questions may have been for rote answers or compliance rather than for offering opinion. Without opportunity for experimenting with query and response, children may not know what they prefer, how to choose, how to inquire, or how to explain.

A child who was hurt for giving the wrong answer may find questions threatening. Questions can be used as an opener to shaming and hurt ("Why do you always have to be such an idiot?" "See what you make me do?"). For some traumatized children, no question is neutral. Being addressed with a question (or being expected to generate one) may bring up feelings of inadequacy, stupidity, inability, vulnerability, anticipation of guilt, helplessness, and pain.

Sarcasm and Humor—What Does Funny Really Mean?

Humor is a learned social skill and part of how we use communication (Bell et al 1986, Halla 1999, Ninio & Snow 1996). Even infants interact through humor. They repeat what makes others laugh in order to elicit the reaction in them, and 'jumpstart' their own laughter to request that silliness be repeated. They begin to laugh with the mere anticipation of what's funny. Funny is most often learned from the reactions of others, and while some interpretation of what's silly may be idiosyncratic (e.g. the YouTube baby who found the sound of tearing paper hilarious), others' responses reinforce or extinguish it. When something is funny, children practice it. They may ask for the same joke repeatedly, enjoying the predictability and familiarity of recognizing the absurd. They 'practice' silliness with their peers, too. They may do silly things together and/or take turns being silly.

Ill, disabled, delayed, and overwhelmed children may have fewer opportunities to engage in humorous exchanges (Suits et al 2011, Rogers & Williams 2006). Some may see people laughing amongst themselves but not know what it means, or not see very much laughter or humor at all (e.g. if growing up with a depressed caregiver). These children can be slow to 'get jokes' or identify what's silly. They may not be good at doing silly things and may not know what to do or that they are expected to laugh. Some may 'try too hard' and go too far, appearing socially clumsy and insensitive. For some abused children, laughter may be very far from funny if they have experience with having been laughed at rather than with. Laughter may be associated with pain and ridicule rather than connection and pleasure, and seeing others laugh can be alarming and remind the child of times when caregivers were drunk, high, or cruel.

Nelly grew up under the care of her paternal aunt, who was often drunk by midday. She learned to stay out of her aunt's way, especially when the aunt's friends—also alcoholics—were around, or risk being the butt of cruel jokes and 'tricks.' The adults treated the child as if she were a circus pet. Their idea of recreation was to add hot sauce to Nelly's chocolate milk, tickle her until she could not breathe, or convince her to attempt things she could not manage. Somehow they found the child's dismay hilarious, and if she cried, they chided her for being a 'spoilsport' and 'too sensitive.' At school, Nelly was suspicious and aggressive. She did not get along well with her peers and often got angry at children who giggled, whether they were directing their mirth at her or not. She herself laughed at children who were crying or upset. "Her laughter sets my teeth on edge," the teacher admitted. "It is more cackle than laughter, really."

Communication Failure: Identifying, Managing, and Responding to Misunderstandings

How one responds to communication failure depends on what one believes one can do about it and what the environment would do in response. Much of it depends on experiences we had with others trying to understand us when we were young and did not yet have many ways of explaining (Cozolino 2006, 2014, van der Kolk 2014). Caregivers often try to interpret a baby's cry or fussiness even through some trial and error. When caregivers remain attuned to the baby's needs, the infant learns to trust that communications matter.

Misunderstandings require repair strategies: We can repeat what we just said so that others have another opportunity to hear it. We can rephrase or clarify by emphasizing what we think was misinterpreted. Whatever we do, the underlying expectation is that the listener is interested in fixing the miscommunication and will use what we offer to help comprehend what we meant; we trust that the communication can be repaired. Repair is reciprocal, and even before they can speak, babies can be active participants in managing misunderstandings. They can cry or cry louder, make faces, smile, fuss, screech, gurgle, cuddle, calm. Babies who experienced many successful interactions are likely to trust their caregivers to fix misinterpretations, and caregivers who usually understand the child feel confident in their abilities to resolve occasional failure. The calm assurance of caregivers also helps children tolerate mild frustrations as they learn to trust that interactions will succeed.

Miscommunications are often less rewarding for maltreated children, who may have had less opportunity with sensitive interactions, less instances of repaired misunderstanding, and more exposure to communication failure. Children may not be asked for input, may be forbidden to 'talk back' or question others, and may not know to repair communication. Furthermore, trauma itself is often incomprehensible and leaves children with overwhelming experiences that remain beyond words or understanding. If confusion is associated with overwhelm, then dissociation and avoidance may be how a child copes with even neutral misunderstandings. If children believe that it is their fault if something goes wrong, they might not want to point it out and risk more shame. By not asking for clarification or redirection, children end up repeating errors. People who assume that a child who said nothing is a child who understood can become upset. Some infer that the child is willful, lazy, or not too bright. In reality the child may be communicating his dearth of skills for repairing failure and misunderstanding.

11 Trauma's Impact on Memory, Organization, and Retrieval

Memory

Memory includes all the information that is perceived and retained in some way, from momentary snapshots of information to long-term memory. How and what we remember is affected by context, relevance, our connection to the people and event, and levels of physiological and emotional activation (Scaer 2014, van der Kolk 2014). Memory span and strategies vary among individuals, and skills can shift within the same person depending on his or her attention and biological, psychological, and emotional state. Stress and overwhelm affect memory, how it is organized, processed, stored, and retrieved (Brewin 2005, Scaer 2014, van der Kolk 2014).

Language is often used to organize, verbalize, conceptualize, and narrate memory, but memories are not limited to verbal memory or narrative memory. Our bodies remember, too. Narrating an event forms an integrated memory of experience (i.e. declarative memory). However, because processing is dampened under stress, trauma is less likely to be stored as an integrated and/or narrative memory and more likely to be stored as (nondeclarative) procedural memory of unconscious conditioned responses of somatic and sensory experience (Brewin 2005, Scaer 2014, van der Kolk 2014). Dissociation further disrupts memory by fragmenting events so they are stored in bits and snapshots of disjointed experience. Without processing (through body therapies and/or verbally), trauma memories often remain detached, compartmentalized, and noncohesive and are vulnerable to being triggered by trauma reminders (Gaensbauer 2011, Howell 2011, Levine & Maté 2010, Siegel 2012, Silberg 2013, Wieland 2011, van der Kolk 2014).

Children's memory, regulatory skills, and language are all still developing, and for them, use of dissociation can affect not only the memory of an experience, but the very way memories are stored and related to. Because overwhelm affects memory storage and retrieval, traumatized children remember events, words, and new and old learning in the way their systems learned to encode them. Sitting in school in states of arousal and hypervigilance (or in numbed dissociation), they cannot remember in the way that nonstressed children can (Cole et al

2005, Yehuda 2005). Tired, hungry, worried, angry, frightened, anxious children cannot remember instruction very well, either. When called to draw on memory (frequent in all learning), chronically traumatized children may respond differently than their peers, in part because they are less able to regulate stress, and even their 'relative calm' can be more activated than that of nontraumatized children (Cole et al 2005, Siegel 2012, Silberg 2013, Wieland 2011). Trauma reminders put them at risk for continued activation that will further affect their processing, remembering, learning, and retrieval. Teachers and caregivers of traumatized children often complain that the children 'don't remember' as they should and have difficulty connecting new information to what was previously taught (Pearce & Pezzot-Pearce 1997, Putnam 1997, Silberg 1998, Yehuda 2004, 2005, 2011).

Context-Dependent Language

Organizing information relies on memory, as knowledge and experience are multilayered and multiply associated. Incoming information is processed to discern whether it repeats, completes, expands, elaborates, or contradicts information we already have. Even when information is completely novel, it becomes connected via associations of time, place, sound, context, person, etc., to other data. How well we process and organize information—and how efficiently we retrieve it later—depends on the way information gets stored to begin with (Brewin 2005, Scaer 2014, van der Kolk 2014). For example, when we recall hearing a speech, the emotions we felt about the situation, the speaker, or the topic, along with smells, noises, or visuals from that time, can all serve as reminders for the event or parts of it. This multisensory processing and organization allows our psyche to retain and integrate information across varied sensations and associations. Trauma disrupts this integrative process. Some sensory, affective, and physiological information can become highlighted and sensitized, while other aspects may be experienced as detached, unreal, or not consciously remembered (Scaer 2014, van der Kolk 2014). Dissociation further disrupts integration of cohesive memory, and while sensory input still gets experienced and reminders (i.e. triggers) can still activate it, the information can surface chaotically and flood the person with sensations, feelings, and physiological responses that can seem completely out of context (Brewin 2005, Gaensbauer 2002, 2011, Howell 2011, Silberg 2013).

In children who experience chronic trauma, processing under stress can become the 'default' way of storing and organizing information. This combination of physiological overwhelm and suppressed access to the 'glue' that language and narrative offer leaves the child susceptible to flooding by trauma reminders and unable to explain or understand what is taking place (Silberg 2013, Wieland 2011). The very act of remembering can become potentially triggering, and certain places, people, things, smells, tastes, and actions can become overwhelming, further reinforcing memory fragmentation and shut down (Gaensbauer 2011, Howell 2011, Levine & Kline 2007, Perry & Szalavitz 2006, van der Kolk 2014). When language (words, phrases, tone) is part of a traumatizing event, listening and language itself can serve as a trauma reminder and trigger memories as well as the emotions, sensations, and dissociation that the trauma elicited.

"My Memory Is Holes"—Jamal: Fragmentation of Memory Processing and Retrieval

Jamal loved school. It was his haven—a parallel universe to life where the nine-year-old rotated with his mother and four younger siblings through the shifting casts of relatives' homes. He rarely had a private corner or knew where he would sleep—whenever his mother outlived the hospitality of wherever they were 'visiting,' they moved on, sometimes in the middle of the night. This usually followed his mother taking off and stranding people with her children, and Jamal both missed her and dreaded her return. Much as Jamal adored school, he was rarely ready for class. When teachers found undone homework in his bag, he would shyly state: "I forgot." Jamal forgot a lot.

Jamal was sweet and unpredictable: sometimes 'on', sometimes 'off,' and his 'memory issues' frustrated the teachers. He could write a page about what they'd just read in social studies but not produce two sentences to a writing prompt like "My favorite TV show is . . ." or "On the weekend I like to . . ." The boy would shrug that he did not remember or would 'borrow' another child's narrative. He could recite what they did in science but 'not remember' what he had for dinner.

Jamal's life appeared compartmentalized: school in one world, home in another. I wondered if he managed the chaos of his home life by having it so that when at school, home did not exist; and when at home, school didn't. His reality fed into the dichotomy: His mother never attended school meetings, and the school apparently did not know that Jamal and his siblings were essentially homeless. Compartmentalization helped Jamal keep the anxieties of home at bay while he was at school, but it also became a liability. To keep the 'two worlds' separate exacted a price when school—his one place of consistency—also became a place of failure and frustration and he was just barely keeping up. "I'm not good at learning," he sighed to me one day. "My memory is holes."

Remembering Not to Remember

Segregating awareness takes energy. It is also imperfect, because trauma reminders 'leak' and intrude anyway, adding stress and unpredictability (Attias & Goodwin 1999, Herman 1997, Scaer 2014, van der Kolk 2014). Triggers are especially scary for children, who often do not understand what is happening or why. An aspect of memory is to be able to differentiate now from then: separating what is being remembered and what took place already from things experienced in the now. However, traumatic memories often superimpose the past onto the present (i.e. flashbacks) having a child feel like it is happening all over again (Silberg 1998, 2013, Waters 2005, Wieland 2011, Yehuda 2011). Remembering does not feel like memory; it feels like now. It makes the bad stuff happen again. To not remember becomes part of surviving.

Children can go to great lengths to not remember trauma, pretend it did not happen, and believe it was unreal (Levine & Kline 2007, Silberg 2013, Wieland 2011). As they work to suppress what is too much to know, chunks of what they do need to know and remember get swept away as well. Whenever triggers inevitably slip through and flood the children with traumatic overwhelm, the children might clamp down further—widening the 'no go zones' in their awareness as they try to contain memory to prevent anxiety (Ford & Courtois 2013, Kluft 1985, Perry & Szalavitz 2006, Silberg 1998, 2013). To remember that there is something scary to forget is scary, too; so children may not be aware of what they push away—they have amnesia to their amnesia—they forget that they forgot.

Understanding the impact of trauma on memory can help place traumatized children's responses and difficulties in context. If remembering things is scary, a child may have less access to academic information and pleasant memories, too. Continued activation also means that children do not learn how to remember well, with even 'good stuff' being stored in ways that are more difficult to recall. What is remembered can come up disjointed, reinforcing confusion and anxiety that then makes further processing difficult. It is a vicious cycle.

"Like a Jigsaw Puzzle in My Brain"—Aggie

"I don't know how to do it!" Ten-year-old Aggie pushed the book away.

"It's the same as what we did yesterday," the teacher tried to be patient. "I showed you how to do it. This is exactly like yesterday."

"I don't remember!" Aggie shook her head in indignation.

The rest of the class barely stirred. Aggie often whined about not knowing how to do something or complained that she was never taught it. The teacher sighed and moved to help another student. She knew that to push Aggie further could agitate the girl further into becoming aggressive. "She's a crack baby," the teacher explained when I began working with Aggie. "Has attention deficit. Lots of behavior issues. Stubborn as they come."

Aggie had to be stubborn. Everything was hard for her. Her attention wavered, and her short-term memory was fickle. By the time the teacher finished giving a direction, Aggie would forget what the direction was about. Even when she tried very hard, she still made errors, and frustration only worsened her focus. Between neurological hypersensitivity from drug exposure and the overwhelming realities she survived, Aggie had plenty of reasons to find remembering difficult.

Aggie was born addicted to cocaine. Prenatal exposure to cocaine is associated with developmental issues, including attention, concentration, memory, and emotional regulation issues (Barth et al 2000, Martin & Dombrowski 2008). Aggie also passed through half a dozen foster-homes between birth and age three, followed by three years of stable fostering before she was temporarily returned to her mother's care. From birth to six, Aggie rarely saw her mother, and then always in supervised visitations where her mother would be on her best behavior. When the mother convinced the court of her sobriety and completion of parenting classes, Aggie lost the one stability she ever had (i.e. her foster-placement) and moved to live with her mother and a younger sibling who had lived with an aunt and whom Aggie barely knew. The change alone was overwhelming, but then the mother revisited old friends and older habits. There were indications that the mother brought men home 'for drug money' and often left the children alone. When Aggie was eight, she had to call for help because her mother was too drugged to rouse. Children's services returned the girls to foster-care and the mother's custody was terminated.

If there was a silver lining, it was that Aggie was returned to the same foster-home that had been her lifeline from age three to six, but she was by no means unscathed. When I met the child two years later, Aggie was eligible for adoption, but her trust had been severely shaken. She wanted to have a 'forever family,' but there were too many disappointments and she was enough of a veteran of the system to realize that her wishes were the smallest part of the equation. She pushed both the past and the future into oblivion, forgetting much else in the bargain.

One day Aggie and I were putting together the story of the class's recent visit to the Bronx Zoo, which I chaperoned. Aggie had taken photos of the animals and we had marked the zoo map with numbered arrows to show our progress. She was able to recall a couple of anecdotes but forgot many others. We had spoken about memory numerous times: how sometimes kids remember only bits here and there if there is too much going on to hold the whole story; how some things can be too confusing to understand. Aggie understood this viscerally. "It is like a jigsaw puzzle in my brain," she frowned, squinting at the map. "It is pieces, and I can't remember; like I am nowhere."

How Can You Recall if You Were Not There? Overwhelm, Dissociation, and Information Inaccessibility

Imagine having a big box where all receipts and documents of several years are meant to be stored. Now visualize yourself on the phone with a service person for the fridge you do not remember buying, yet need to produce the proof of purchase for. Riffling frantically through the box, you have no idea what the receipt looks like or if it is even there. You certainly do not remember putting it there because you are not sure you even bought the fridge, though the person on the other end of the line states you had. As your mind scrambles to try and remember what you do not recall or what the heck it means that you cannot remember it, this receipt searching is likely to be stressful—let alone if you keep stumbling across all manner of things you had no idea about or forgot to take care of.... Your distress is likely to escalate if failing to unearth the document will have repercussions (i.e. no service and your holiday food ruined). Even if you manage to find the receipt, the anxiety around it will have made the whole episode unsettling and you might never want to see that box (or fridge) again: The very presence of it may be too distressing.

When memory is unreliable—due to inability, lack of processing, or dissociation—it can be confusing and frustrating to try and access what one knows or should know. That is reality for many children with language-processing and retrieval issues, along with children who endure overwhelm (Bellis 2002, Brinton & Fujiki 1989, Cohen 2001, Cole et al 2005, Cross 2004, Danon-Boileau 2002, Fox et al 1988, Heymann 2010, Hilyard & Wolfe 2002, Kurtz et al 1993, Kuttner 2010, Nadeau & Polin 2013, McAleer-Hamaguchi 2001, Perez & Widom 1994, Putnam 1993, Shirar 1996, Schaefer et al 1991, Yehuda 2011). When information is ineffectively processed and stored, some of it can be completely missed. Children may not realize they missed things until they fail or do not know what is expected. They often cannot explain why: They do not remember not remembering. Like the box of documents, the very situation of being asked a question can become stressful, with anxiety then making things harder to remember, reinforcing stress and shame.

The ability of traumatized children to learn can shift with the level of stress they are experiencing at the moment. This often does not match the stress others believe there is to feel: what can seem a perfectly calm setting to caregivers and teachers may not feel that way to the child (Silberg 2013, Wieland 2011). Hypervigilance and dissociation affect learning not only at the time of learning but later on as well, because the information may not be accessible if it was learned when the child was stressed. A child may tune out something in class due to trauma reminders or distress, only to be faced with questions on it in her homework. When the homework itself brings up anxiety, the child may tune out the very fact that there is homework and then the teacher's scolding, too. A child may not remember why others are angry at him, and feel upset that he is being punished for something he never knew he had to do.

"I Never Get a Turn!"—Ralph: When Memory Escapes Reality

Ralph spent more time in detention than in his classroom. The fifth grader was aggressive and distracting. Taller than me and twice as heavy, the boy could (and did) inflict serious damage to property and people when mad—throwing tables across the room and smashing chairs against the wall. Teachers and students feared his strength and hair-trigger fury. All I knew of Ralph's history was that his father was in jail with a long rap sheet, much of it violent. Rumor had it that the boy stepped between his father and his mother several times and got knocked out cold once in the process.

When not raging, Ralph was huffy and silent at the back of the class (to not block other students' view) fiddling with this or that and rarely seeming to pay attention. Then his face would redden, the veins in his neck would swell, and he would push away from his desk. It was like watching thunderclouds—you knew a storm was coming and all you could do was try to find shelter and hope for the best. Small things upset him: someone popping their knuckles, the screeching of car wheels outside, some tones of voices. He would get angry when he wanted to answer and another student was called, and could explode in indignation even if he just had a turn. "It's not fair!" he would bellow, pushing his desk away. "Not fair! I never get a turn!"

After some violent outbursts, the school's protocol was that if Ralph even began to get upset the teacher was to summon the security officer, conveniently positioned just down the hall. Ralph was big, but that man was far bigger. His appearance alone often took the wind out of Ralph's sails, and the boy deflated and sat down. Other times Ralph remained standing, his back to the wall in more ways than one. The security officer would step into the room, making it clear that he would bodily remove the boy if needed. Witnessing this once, I could not help but wonder about the likely similarities (read: reenactment) between the security officer and Ralph's dad.

"Ralph, you need to go with Mr. Karson and get yourself under control," the teacher had noted as Ralph glared. A few seconds of stand-off ensued. The children nearest to Ralph remained vigilant, but others watched curiously or ignored the whole thing. The boy remained standing defiantly and the security officer walked over, towered above him, grabbed Ralph's arm above the elbow, and stated: "Let's go." Ralph let himself be led. Even before the boy's wide back disappeared into the hall, the class continued as if nothing had happened. It was eerie and sad.

I often found Ralph in the detention room. The lumbering eleven-year-old would sit dejected and quiet, fiddling with his pencil, ignoring the one or two other banished students. The detention-room teacher, an older guy of few words and even fewer facial expressions, kept the children at significant wingspan from each other, rarely spoke to the children, and did not acknowledge their distress if they were crying or mumbling in ire. His apathy unsettled me, but maybe his few demands felt familiar or gave the children space to regroup in whatever way they knew how. Ralph—or the others—were often asleep, staring, or rocking their chairs back from the desks, trying to balance life.

For all his fury at the constant banishing, I believe Ralph used the detention room to regroup. Unfortunately, it meant more missed instruction, which back-fired in frustration and more banishment. There was very little space for Ralph to communicate with the classroom teacher—any hint of reactivity meant being sent out—and the nonexistent tolerance for his affect only reinforced his polarized behavior. He was either 'checked out' or 'kicked out.'

Ralph needed help with vocabulary, comprehension, reading, problem solving, word problems, and narrative. He could not catch up when he was effectively not in class, physically or otherwise. Even in session, Ralph could flicker in and out of connection, and his participation was disjointed. His responses could be breathtakingly relevant; other times, not so much. He was actually a quick learner: When engaged, he caught on fast and could be quite animated when he wasn't in a huff. Then something—a noise, a cloud shifting the light, an error—would have him shift to anger or shut down. He was never aggressive with me, but by the time he managed to get grounded he would find it difficult to remember what he learned, forget the words, claim he was never shown them; just as in class he would demand a turn when he just had one . . .

Trauma and dissociation do not affect all children's school performance, ability, and behavior similarly. Some struggle across the board. Some manage surprisingly well in spite of fragmented awareness. Some become excellent readers of other people, tell them what they want to hear, and manage to fly under the radar regardless of their skill levels. Some speak very little. Some speak eloquently. Some speak too much. Some disengage, some cling. There is no one clinical profile to describe all traumatized children and no one presentation that would single out who was or was not overwhelmed. Nevertheless there are some things clinicians can remain alert to; communication profiles that can serve as red flags for overwhelm as a possible contributing factor. Recognizing those—and reacting in ways that validate the broken places—may help minimize the times where we end up missing the communications of children who need so desperately to be heard.

Part 4

When Communication Goes Awry

Clinical Presentation and
Assessment Challenges

12 Communication Symptoms in Traumatized and Dissociative Children

As described in previous chapters, trauma places children at high risk for communication issues due to the effects of overwhelm and dissociation on development, learning, and relating (Fox et al 1988, Pearce & Pezzot-Pearce 1997, Silberg 1998, Yehuda 2005). In addition, children who already have disabilities and/or primary communication disorders can be further impacted by stress and maltreatment (Benedict et al 1990, Cappadocia et al 2011, Crosse et al 1993, Goldson 1998, Hershkowitz et al 2007, Sullivan et al 1991, 2009). Whenever a child has a history of trauma, assessing communication issues is important. It is also crucial to be on the lookout for trauma components in any children with communication disorders, because of their increased risk for trauma and maltreatment. Even when a communication disorder is not evident, one should be alert to difficulties in processing, pragmatics, attending, learning, and relating.

Some aspects of communication difficulties seen in traumatized children (e.g. small vocabularies) are similar to those in children with 'regular' language-learning issues. In many children these difficulties indeed overlap with existing communication disorders (Sullivan et al 1991, 2009), and maltreated children are twice as likely to require special education (Cole et al 2005, Pearce & Pezzot-Pearce 1997, Putnam 1997). Other clinical aspects can seem atypical or inconsistent or cluster in ways that can serve as red flags to the presence of overwhelm from maltreatment, trauma, or the child's experiences of distress. This chapter will summarize the communication presentation that can be seen in traumatized children. It will briefly revisit trauma-sensitive language aspects (described at length in Part 3) and offer possible explanations for how a child's clinical picture may reflect his/her particular reality.

Prevalence studies in maltreated and traumatized children describe them as tending to be literal, with short attention spans, small vocabularies, and low school performance. Their responses to emotion-evoking pictures can be ambiguous, and they can have deficits in discourse (Attias & Goodwin 1999, Pearce & Pezzot-Pearce 1997, Putnam 1993, 1997, Yehuda 2005, 2011). They tend to have simplified repetitive play, cause classroom disturbance, repeat grades, and show poor ability to maintain involvement, along with aggression and social incompetence (Pearce & Pezzot-Pearce 1997, Putnam 1997, Silberg 1998, 2013, Yehuda 2004, 2005, 2011). Traumatized children can have inconsistent skills and behaviors and are often diagnosed with ADD/ADHD, bipolar disorder, OCD, ODD, autism, and other diagnoses (Cole et al 2005, Miller 2005, Waters 2005, Silberg 1998, 2013).

Language Content, Use, and Symbolic Play

Semantic Issues—Body-State Language, Affective Words

Maltreated children tend to have smaller expressive vocabularies than nonmal-treated children and can struggle to express themselves verbally (Pearce & Pezzot-Pearce 1997, Putnam 1997, Yehuda 2005). While many children with language impairment present with limited expressive vocabularies, traumatized children often have certain areas of vocabulary that are especially affected. These include body-state language (e.g. hungry, tired, cold) and emotional/affective language (e.g. sad, worried, happy, anxious), which can be disproportionately impacted compared with less personal lexical items. For some traumatized children, certain sensory modalities or semantic contexts may appear especially problematic, possibly reflecting the child's specific trauma and coping. For example, a child may show a markedly different semantic ability (or use) for visual descriptors compared with auditory or tactile descriptors, perhaps mirroring avoidance of visual trauma reminders and/or coping that involved 'shutting down' visual processing to 'not see' or 'not remember' overwhelming things.

Cause-Effect and Sequence Issues

Understanding and describing sequence is often difficult for traumatized children as it includes identifying how one thing leads to the next, as well as explaining the chain of events—aspects of reality that trauma often disrupts. Traumatized children may struggle to predict the ending of a story or the consequences of (theirs or others') actions. They may come up with idiosyncratic and unexpected explanations for events or predictions for what may happen next (e.g. 'Why is the child smiling when opening a present?' "Because she going to cry" or "No one brung her any." 'What may happen if the milk spills?' "He going to be very cold").

While sequence may be difficult for many children with language impairment, this area can appear especially affected in traumatized children. It may not match a child's overall ability and can be particularly affected in interpersonal language or specific contexts. Causation and sequence can be elusive for a child who was hit regardless of misbehavior, or is confused by why painful medical interventions happened even 'when they were good.' Children's interpretation of causation can reflect their beliefs, confusion, and overwhelm. In addition, overwhelm affects processing and integration so that perception of causation and sequence may be fragmented, with events appearing to take place in a disconnected way. Such fragmentation may be present in certain contexts or extend into many scenarios and may reflect a child's dissociation and level of confusion about how things interrelate or cause each other.

Some children show an overall understanding of causation and sequence but struggle to apply it in some topics (i.e. maybe those that elicit stress or associate with trauma reminders). They may describe some sequences well and fail miserably on others. In older children, fluctuations can seem more subtle, presenting in differences in the child's ability to apply skills to fiction versus nonfiction analysis, to certain topics, or in unusual inferences about intent, motive, and causation in characters' actions and predictions of outcome.

Temporal Concepts

Temporal concepts are related to sequence, and because they are relative and ambiguous they may be particularly confusing. Conveying time and temporal order requires mentally organizing events in a sequence and having sufficient expressive ability to 'walk someone through' the event from start to finish. Children with communication disorders often struggle with comprehension and application of "before/after," "yesterday/last week," "first/then," "meanwhile/during/following," etc. Temporal concepts are exquisitely vulnerable to overwhelm (Terr 1983), and traumatized children's difficulties with these concepts can highlight other language and communication aspects that are impacted by trauma.

If a child misses parts of events because she 'zoned out' or was hypervigilant, it can be hard for her to understand the order of things. Not only does dissociation disrupt perceptions of "during" and "afterward," but trauma reminders themselves can make it feel like the trauma is happening again. This can make it difficult to comprehend (or explain) the difference between before/after, happening/over, now/then. Trauma time does not move in one direction only: The past invades the present and things from before overlap things from now, making time confusing.

In addition, the very perception of time can be altered during trauma. People report time 'standing still' or 'stretching' during traumatizing events. Some experience the world 'moving in slow motion' or 'being distorted' (Terr 1983). Continued overwhelm can distort time even more, let alone if one's time concepts are still evolving, as they are in children. Time concepts can be tricky for young children, let alone when time itself becomes intrinsically connected to the trauma and/or the anticipation of it. Even children without understanding of clocks can associate event proximities (e.g. Daddy will come home after you have dinner). In traumatized children, proximities can be terrifying (e.g. burns scrubbed every day after nursing changes). Children may form associations that feel temporally related (e.g. Mom brought pizza and a painful thing took place, so pizza time means pain). Such idiosyncratic interpretation can be very difficult for adults to decipher or a child to explain, especially if the concept of time is still evolving or if the child has no words for it or fears verbalizing it lest the bad things happen again.

Narrative

Trauma disrupts narrative, and narrative ability in maltreated children can appear immature (Kluft 1985, Pearce & Pezzot-Pearce 1997, Putnam 1997). It can also seem inconsistent, with the child narrating well sometimes, then poorly at other times (Yehuda 2005). Personal narrative may be especially impacted. Children can find it difficult to tell events that involve themselves or their experiences. Their affect may be dull, incongruent, or odd, and they may focus on trivial aspects of events or stories instead of forming a coherent narrative with feelings and interactions, a beginning, middle, and end.

Sometimes difficulties with narrative represent shifts in children's level of awareness during the event they are trying to narrate. If they 'checked out' for part of it, what they manage to tell may indeed be choppy and noncohesive. Other times fluctuations in narrative quality may reflect the child's difficulty with the content or the association of an event, or the trauma reminders it evokes. The context does not have to be overtly upsetting or outwardly dramatic for it to associate with overwhelming aspects of trauma, which are often intertwined with the mundane (e.g. eating soup if that was when Dad hit Mom, or when the pot tipped and they got burned). Fluctuations can be especially telling if children begin narrating cohesively and then shift to a noncohesive, affectless, or odd narrative.

Difficulties in causation, sequence, temporal concepts, description, or narrative are not in and of themselves specific to or singularly indicative of trauma. However, when taken into account alongside other aspects of communication, a child's language and behavior across various contexts is important information. Language provides insight into the child's perceptions and can offer input about assumptions about the world and people in it, and is informative both when the child is able and unable to describe them.

"Access" and Retrieval Issues

There are many reasons why traumatized children can appear at a loss for words for describing experiences. Difficulty 'accessing' words is common in children with language impairments and word-retrieval issues (i.e. having words 'on the tip of the tongue'). Traumatized children encounter similar difficulties that may appear disproportionately worse for particular aspects or contexts (e.g. affective words, talking about home). Most children with retrieval issues have some contexts they find easier, better days and not so great ones, and can find it harder to retrieve under stress. However, these fluctuations can be more pronounced in traumatized children (and in children with both communication disorders and trauma). Children may show retrieval issues one day but very little difficulty the next, or have drastic changes in retrieval within a very short span of time (e.g. a session), which may be associated with certain contexts, people, or internal states that elicit stress (Kluft 1985, Silberg 1998, 2013, Waters 2005, Wieland 2011). Because trauma affects processing, memory, and organizing of information, trauma reminders (and their associations) can make formulating thoughts on certain topics difficult (Brewin 2005, Cozolino 2014, Gaensbauer 2011, Scaer 2014, van der Kolk 2014).

Pragmatics: Social Cues, Turn-Taking, Humor, and Metaphor

Trauma affects interaction and can disrupt social relatedness and the way language is used. It can limit children's pragmatic ability and distort their experience with certain pragmatic cues. Chronic trauma derails many relational and developmental processes, and communication can be especially affected because of the way stress dampens processing and language access (Siegel 2012, van der Kolk 2014). Children with developmental trauma can be overly passive (reacting versus initiating interaction) or overly aggressive ('hogging' the stage, not listening, ignoring others' social cues) or seem unaware of discourse rules (Kluft 1985, Pearce & Pezzot-Pearce 1997, Putnam 1997, Silberg 1998, 2013, Vissing et al 1991, Wieland 2011, Yehuda 2005, 2011). Some appear lost when it comes to taking turns or keeping on topic, may behave crassly or seem to lack empathy. They can be clumsy with humor, not knowing when to laugh or what to laugh about, laugh too loudly or too long, or at things others do not find funny (e.g. a crying child). These behaviors often 'earn' the children a reputation as antisocial, oppositional, and autistic (Briscoe-Smith & Hinshaw 2006, Jamora et al 2009, Miller 2005, Rogers & Williams 2006, Scherr 2007, Smith et al 1998, Yehuda 2005, 2011). Their behavior may represent the rules a child derived from his/her experiences. It is important to look at children's behaviors through the lens of their history and to pay close attention to whether issues manifest more in certain contexts or with certain people.

Symbolic Play and Imagination

Traumatized children—especially young ones—may not know how to play. They may use items stereotypically rather than symbolically and use repetitive rather than creative play (Putnam 1997, Silberg 1998, 2013). Some play appropriately but with a very narrow repertoire. What can appear stereotypical, repetitive, or narrow may provide a peek into the child's reality: the little boy who hid all the adult toy figures; the girl who kept dislocating the 'mommy' doll's arms; the kindergartener whose range of symbolic play was sitting the dolls on the chairs, feeding them, and putting them to bed; the preschooler who constantly 'packed suitcases.'

Trauma and overwhelm affect a child's availability for healthy imagination and creative play (Blanc et al 2005, Kaminski et al 2002, Kluft 1985, Kuttner 2010, Landy & Menna 2001, Schaefer et al 1991, Silberg 1998). Some traumatized children use too little imagination. Others use too much or may find it difficult to use imagination on demand (e.g. creative writing, social role-play). Some are literal and confront others' imaginary play ("Why you lying? Dogs can't talk," "I can't be the fireman, that's not a real hose," "This is all stupid made-up stuff"). Then there are the children who spend most of their time in imaginary places and may find it difficult to shift from imaginary play to everyday reality; the 'space cadets' who miss much of what goes on around them. Some children rigidly play one or two imaginary themes (e.g. playing 'police,' having everything 'dog related') and become anxious or refuse to elaborate or change them. This makes them 'not fun' for peers to play with and reduces their opportunities for play and healthy interaction. For children who depend on mentally escaping into their minds to survive, imagination can become both refuge and desert island.

Skill Fluctuation and Amnesia

Lying

The line between imagination and lying can be tricky for children: It is okay to pretend you are Superman or a princess but it is not okay to pretend you did not eat your brother's cookie; Daddy can be the horse and you can be the sheriff but neither is actually true; it is okay to wrestle in pretend but if you get angry and hit someone for real, you can't say it was only pretend even if it happened in a game. The boundary between truth and falsehood can be especially tricky for traumatized children escaping into fantasy. It can also be difficult for those confused about what happened or those who experienced outright lies regarding what did or did not happen or was done to them. Maltreated children may appear to lie a lot. If you pretended to be someplace else whenever Daddy yelled at Mommy, did it make it not really happen? If Mom says "Stop lying, I did not hit you" when your face still hurts, did you only imagine her hitting you? Was it pretend? Is she lying? Are you lying? What does it mean to deny that something happened? Does it make it not be?

Dissociation (and its close cousin, amnesia) complicates reality further. Children often lie to stay out of trouble, but sometimes a child's denial of misbehavior—especially in the face of obvious evidence—can be indicative of dissociation (Kluft 1985, Silberg 1998, 2013, Waters 2005, Wieland 2011). For children who experience chronic stress or have a trauma history, amnesia should be considered a possibility, because overwhelming affect combined with helplessness often lead to dissociation (Lyons-Ruth et al 2006, van der Kolk 2014). Escaping 'inside their mind' or 'outside of their body' can be the only 'out' a child has. Being 'away' could have events be less available for retrieval or feel less real or as if they did not happen. Children may not remember doing what they are accused of doing. They may seem to be lying when they may not be.

For those children who use dissociation habitually and/or whose life experiences taught them irrational cause-and-effect, consequences can be difficult to understand. They may not see how their actions connect with the results of those actions and may claim innocence when they are guilty. Some appear to "not learn a lesson" or behave "oppositional" and disrespectful of boundaries (Bruning 2007, ISSTD Child and Adolescent Committee 2008, Scherr 2007, Silberg 1998, 2013, Smith et al 1998). In actuality the children's behavior may be a reflection of their reality rather than inherent lack of moral capability, motivation, or empathy.

Lack of Motivation, Denial, and Fluctuations in Ability

Caregivers understandably become frustrated with children who deny misbehavior, refuse to do work, and have 'attitude.' Traumatized children are often described as lacking motivation, stubborn, passive, or 'checked out.' They can appear capable but resistant, simultaneously needy and dismissive (Pearce & Pezzot-Pearce 1997, Putnam 1997, Silberg 1998, Yehuda 2005, 2011). Teachers and caregivers complain that the children are "unwilling to work" or "refuse to do things they know how to do." Traumatized children can be confusing, and the confusion they evoke in others may be mirroring the child's reality and how they learned to cope.

What may seem as an unwillingness to work may reflect dissociation, amnesia, and lack of availability for learning. While traumatized children are certainly capable of manipulating to get out of doing work, ongoing 'resistance' and claims of inability should lead one to consider overwhelm as part of the equation. Forgetfulness and changes in skill level can be especially indicative of stress when they appear in activities a child usually enjoys yet claims to not know how to do or to have forgotten how (Waters 2005, Wieland 2011, Yehuda 2005).

The behavior of all children changes with circumstances, but in traumatized children those shifts can go beyond such everyday variation. In some children, mood, behavior, or abilities shift so abruptly or completely that educators and caregivers state, "Oh, there he goes . . ." when they see the child 'about to get upset' or 'lose interest.' In other children, these shifts can be outwardly subtle but affect function and involvement. We may not always know what can be at the base of fluctuations, but marked changes in a child should raise flags to possible dissociation (Kluft 1985, Silberg 1998, 2013, Waters 2005, Wieland 2011).

'Diagnosis Misfits' and 'Diagnosis Accumulators'

Multiple Diagnoses

Many doctors, psychiatrists, psychologists, and teachers remain unaware of dissociative features in children, and it is common for traumatized and dissociative children to end up with multiple diagnoses, misdiagnoses, and missed diagnoses (Waters 2005, Silberg 2013, Wieland 2011). This may happen even when trauma history is evident (Bruning 2007, Cole et al 2005, Cross 2004, Danon-Boileau 2002, Gray 2002, Smith et al 1998). Adverse events may not be taken into account if time has passed since the trauma and/or the child is believed to be in a safe environment. Trauma history is also unlikely to be included in relation to education and academic instruction, and even children who have marked trauma histories may not have these noted in their individual educational programs (IEPs). Sometimes the only indication a teacher has of a child's adverse life events is the fact the child is in foster-care (i.e. and so at the very least has endured attachment disruption, if not additional trauma in what had led the removal from parental custody).

The high prevalence of maltreatment, and the complex ways children can be exposed to overwhelming stress, should place a high index of suspicion for trauma history as contributing to a child's clinical presentation (US-DHHS 2013a, van der Kolk 2005). Whenever children with communication issues have multiple diagnoses, it is important to look beyond the labels and examine the child's symptoms, behaviors, and responses. This is not to dismiss the validity of diagnoses per se—in fact, many co-occur with trauma, and almost any childhood diagnosis increases the risk for trauma (Benedict et al 1990, Crosse et al 1993, Goldson 1998, Hershkowitz et al 2007, Knutson & Sullivan 1993, Sullivan et al 1987, 1991, 2009). However, an accumulation of diagnoses can also reflect symptoms explainable by developmental trauma (Silberg 1998, 2013, Stolbach et al 2013, Waters 2005, van der Kolk 2005).

Clinical presentation is inherently complex and idiosyncratic. Differential diagnosis is important in any clinical setting, as is the consideration of comorbidity, co-occurrence, and contributing factors. When symptoms worsen, change, or do not quite fit, it is essential to consider what additional factors may be at play to add or complicate ongoing difficulties. Understanding the role of overwhelm (and the coping mechanisms to manage it), along with the impact of trauma on the specific child in his/her specific difficulty constellation, can help elucidate what the child is experiencing. It can also offer ways to identify and minimize the impact of stress on the child, so that benefits of intervention can be maximized and the child's well-being improved.

Masquerade: Look-alike Symptoms, Differential Diagnosis, and Comorbidity

Trauma responses can often masquerade as symptoms of other disorders (Scaer 2014, Silberg 1998, 2013, Waters 2005, van der Kolk 2014). Abuse, hyper-vigilance, dissociation, numbing, and irritability affect a child's ability to attend, but when a child shows difficulty attending, stares into space, and cannot sit still, they are likely to be diagnosed with ADD/ADHD (Attention Deficit/Hyperactivity Disorder) (Briscoe-Smith & Hinshaw 2006, Cole et al 2005, Fuller-Thomson et al 2014). Trauma affects language and processing, but when a child presents with difficulty in expressing ideas, comprehending information, or following directions, they are likely to be diagnosed with a Language Learning Delay, Receptive-Expressive Language Disorder, or Auditory Processing Disorder (Bellis 2002, Cohen 2001, Cross 2004, Danon-Boileau 2002, Heymann 2010). If they exhibit (seemingly) unprovoked aggression, they are likely to be diagnosed with ODD (Oppositional Defiant Disorder) or a Conduct Disorder (Cole et al 2005, Waters 2005, Wieland 2011). Traumatized children may use out-of-context phrasing when triggered and may have incongruent affect, lack of eye-contact, rocking, or shrinking away; behaviors that often lead to a diagnosis of Autism (Danon-Boileau 2002, Miller 2005). Trauma may lead to perseveration-like behaviors, periods of altered presence and amnesia, which may result in diagnosis of neurological or psychotic issues (Danon-Boileau 2002, Netherton et al 1999, Perry & Szalavitz 2006). While the above diagnoses can co-occur with trauma, the possibility of trauma needs to be assessed as well if one is to consider whether symptoms—or some symptoms—are explained by posttraumatic or dissociative symptoms (Cole et al 2005, Kluft 1985, Putnam 1993, 1997, Silberg 1998, 2013, Silva 2004, van der Kolk 2005, Waters 2005, Wieland 2011, Yehuda 2005).

Jason: ADHD or Dissociation?

I met Jason when he was eight. I was warned to "watch out" for his aggression and extreme reactivity: EMS had been called twice to school for "out of control behavior." "His emotions and behavior are on steroids," the teacher stated. The boy oscillated from rage to uncontrolled giggling, aggression, "babyish crying," and "resistant" behavior. He was in constant motion, fidgeting and jumping at every sound, disruptive, impulsive, and seemingly unaware of 'personal space.' He bumped into, pushed past, touched, and grabbed. Jason could not yet read but faked it, using sight words and guessing others from context, and got furious if anyone corrected him. He accused teachers of "making it too hard on purpose" and giving him words he "never seen before." He griped for hours on alleged injustices, weaving together bits of varied events in disjointed 'tirades.'

Teachers and principal believed Jason "must have ADHD" and that "if he paid better attention he could be reading but he doesn't like to work hard, just daydream or fool around." The school counselor claimed Jason was "symptomatically scattered but positive for ADHD" (and oppositional disorder, bipolar disorder, language/learning disorder, and dyslexia). Trauma was not assessed but the counselor pressed: "The boy is fine. His grandma is taking really good care of him."

Jason had lived with his maternal grandmother since age four and a half. Kind but overwhelmed, she supported an older handicapped son, Jason, and another granddaughter she had custody of. Jason's father disappeared before he was born, and his mother was 'found unfit.' Apparently his mother would leave him with relatives "for an hour" but disappear for days. It was also believed that her 'boyfriend' (i.e. pimp) "maybe interfered with the boy." Though mandated for counseling, Jason rarely attended because the school counselor claimed him "too destructive, doesn't sit still, and a bad influence on others in the group."

He was in 1:1 in speech-language therapy, where he was usually calm and tried to participate, becoming upset by particular things rather than "generally uncooperative." Some days Jason was especially on edge (e.g. after visiting his mother in jail, after a fight in the classroom). "I can't get back into myself," he once told me. Spending more time on grounding helped. In class, Jason's teacher agreed to try the 'Tool-Kit' (see Part 5*). It helped curtail 'acting out escalation' and she became attentive to signs of mood shifts, assisting Jason before things got bad. "I'm not sure he has ADHD in my class anymore," she said to me. "He still checks out sometimes if I don't 'catch it' but he calms down when he hears my voice." She smiled sheepishly, "As long as I don't yell. He still checks out on me if I forget and yell . . ."*

Jason lived in his grandmother's relatively stable home for almost half his life, but the shadows of his earlier years were still there. Did Jason have ADHD, or were the attention issues related to hypervigilance? Did he have bipolar disorder, or were his mood shifts reactions to triggers and difficulties in regulation explainable by his early beginnings? Regardless of what diagnoses he might have gotten with a trauma-sensitive assessment, he responded well to grounding, calming, and de-escalation. No longer seeing his shifts as signs of an irascible attitude but as calls for help, his teacher improved their relationship. She saw an endearing side to a student who she previously felt was "testing her." Jason no longer felt she "wanted to get him in trouble."

Dissociation, hypervigilance, and overwhelm can affect emotional shifts and difficulties in regulating them. Because traumatized children may be reacting to personal trauma reminders and internal interpretation of events, they can seem to inexplicably 'swing' from one emotional state to another (Kluft 1985, Silberg 2013, Waters 2005, Wieland 2011). Childhood disorders and disabilities (e.g. ADHD, bipolar disorder, autism) can include difficulties with emotional regulation, which place children at high risk for maltreatment and overwhelm (Briscoe-Smith & Hinshaw 2006, Cappadocia et al 2011, Fuller-Thomson et al 2014, Knutson & Sullivan 1993, Sullivan & Knutson 2000). Even without maltreatment, stress in chronic illness and disability can be exacerbated by repeated failure and difficulty (Carlsson et al 2008, Drew 2007, Kuttner 2010, Johnson & Francis 2005, Ødegård 2005, Varni et al 1996).

Recognizing and understanding the role of stress and coping as part of a child's difficulties is integral to appropriate intervention. The treatment for ADHD or autism is not the same as the treatment for posttraumatic or dissociative issues. For example, therapies that demand eye contact or repetition may be helpful in some cases of autism but can actually reinforce dissociation if the child is trying to disengage as self-protection. It is also important to take into account how communication difficulties affect assessment and how children's stress can impact their presentation and abilities.

Language and Testing Issues in Trauma

The Effect of Trauma on Language Testing

Assessment is at best a snapshot of an individual's ability at a particular moment with the particular tester in the particular setting. When attempting to assess skills, especially in children, clinicians do their best to have it be a fair representation of abilities by minimizing interfering variables or at the very least remaining cognizant of their impact on testing. We understand that due to the impact of malaise on attention, motivation, memory, and interaction, the language of children who are unwell may not represent their actual ability.

Similarly, children who 'employ' posttraumatic coping skills during an assessment may give results that misrepresent their potential. Their performance may be affected by their overall stress level that day or by what got triggered by a question, the setting, or the examiner. It can be impacted by what happened in and out of the room, who accompanied them, what the children understood the testing was for, their interpretation of errors, prior experience with testing, etc. Conclusions from any testing session are partial. They can be even more so in children whose performance was impacted by stress and dissociation, which makes it doubly important that professionals who come into contact with children understand and identify signs of hyperarousal, dissociation, and withdrawal.

Given the reality of how maltreatment and overwhelm affect language and communication, speech-language pathologists (as well as other professionals who assess children) should take careful histories about trauma (see Chapter 13) and remain attuned to children's responses during interactions. Children who responded well to several test items but cannot complete items of similar difficulty may be showing issues with sustaining focus, attention, or fatigue. However, they may also be reacting to something in the content of a test item—this one or the one before the change in behavior, or the lot. It is helpful to take note of the kind of reaction the child had: how abrupt it was, the child's affect, and his response to supportive redirection and grounding. Also, when a child shows an unusual response or a shift in affect and attention, grounding may be needed before testing should be continued. Alternate test questions of equivalent difficulty and varied content (even if it cannot be scored) can help ascertain whether a shift was about skill or content. Such interactions can provide information about how the child responds, reorients, manages errors, and responds to communication failure and repair.

The Effect of Language Issues on Psychological Assessment

Language is integral to counseling. However, unless a child arrived in psychotherapy with an already diagnosed language delay or disorder, many psychotherapists working with traumatized and dissociative children assume normal language skills (at least for nontrauma material). When children provide non–age appropriate or incongruent responses, psychotherapists can misunderstand those as reflecting psychological or thought disorders rather than language issues or communication difficulties. In order to minimize misreading of children's actual abilities or underlying issues, it is important that psychotherapists understand the impact of language and communication issues on assessment and intervention.

Rating scales. Rating scales provide a quick way to assess whether a child falls within a normal range emotionally and behaviorally. Scoring predetermined sets of questions can help clinicians discern whether a child or adolescent tests positive for depression, anxiety, compulsion, and so on. Even though many children with behavioral-emotional issues also have language impairments, rating scales are rarely calibrated for children with communication and language delays. When rating scales were used with children who had speech-language impairment, the results were skewed to over-identify socioemotional disorders (Redmond 2002).

Clinical interviews. Designed to help gather information flexibly through open-ended questions while establishing rapport and trust, clinical interviews can be vulnerable to language limitations. Communication issues can affect not only the content of children's replies but also how well they comprehended the questions, as well as how the children (or adolescents) conveyed information and how they interpreted or responded to lack of understanding.

Projective techniques/tasks. Communication issues can impact the results of projective techniques. Projective tasks assume comprehension of directions and carry implicit linguistic demands for things like fluent retrieval of words, production of complex syntax, interpretation of figurative language or symbolic representation, and understanding of temporal concepts. All these depend heavily on language skills, vocabulary skills, processing skills, retrieval skills, and narrative skills, which are vulnerable to communication and language issues.

Assessment measures are helpful. It is only that one should use the results with awareness of how language and communication may affect and be affected by content, context, and interpretation. Children with developmental, emotional, and communication disorders are at higher risk for trauma, and traumatized children are at risk for having developmental, emotional, and communicative impacts to relating, learning, socializing, and growing. This creates a tricky but rich diagnostic landscape, where clinicians are called to consider various factors and weigh their relative impacts to reach a 'good enough' diagnosis that explains current symptoms and charts a path to treatment. To do so, we need to be aware of the interplay of trauma, communication, and development, along with the physiological and psychological vulnerabilities of the child or adolescent. Access to sufficient information, along with knowing what to ask and recognizing what we see and hear (or what is withheld), are important aspects for achieving that.

13 History, Screening, and Assessment Indicators

Trauma History—Not 'Just' about Overt Abuse

Maltreatment is and remains a very significant cause of trauma in children. However, as detailed in Part 2, maltreatment is not the only cause of trauma in children. Medical trauma (prematurity, interuterine exposure to substances, congenital issues, chronic illness and chronic pain, accidents and invasive procedures), war trauma, exposure to violence, refugee status, overwhelmed or ill caregivers, loss and separation can also be sources of trauma in children and affect their clinical presentation.

Assessment requires that we incorporate much information in a short time, trying to gather developmental, medical, neurological, relational, communicative, and social information, all while creating rapport with an adult and a child and testing different skills (Brinton & Fujiki 1989, Gleason & Ratner 2009, Piazza & Carroll-Hernandez 2004, Schiefelbusch 1986, Schaefer et al 1991). There are questions one should not ask in the presence of a child. Also, it may not be possible to cover everything within the timeframe of a single assessment, and assessment often continues in some form throughout intervention. That said, whenever possible, there are data worth inquiring about prior to the evaluation itself and/or keeping in mind for follow-up:

- Prenatal stressors (maternal physical and/or emotional difficulties during the pregnancy: loss and grief, trauma, domestic issues, medications, and exposures to substances)
- Postnatal and infancy stressors (difficulties during labor, complications, stay in the neonatal intensive care unit (NICU) and what it entailed, colic and reflux, parental stress and availability, postpartum depression, caregiver illness, domestic and economic stressors, caregiver consistency, attachment difficulties)
- Medical history (surgeries and hospitalizations, accidents, invasive procedures, medications, ear infections, respiratory issues like asthma, and chronic conditions and what their management entails)
- Developmental issues (growth and achievement of motor and developmental milestones, sleep patterns and feeding patterns, temperament and ease of

soothing, sensory sensitivities, alertness and engagement, communication patterns, self-soothing behaviors, unusual habits or needs)
- Familial history (sibling issues; illness and disabilities; family configuration and stability; domestic stressors—violence, separations, or custody issues; chronic illness or chronic pain in caregivers; trauma history in caregivers; mental illness in caregivers or close family members)
- Environmental stressors (economic issues—loss of job, work pressure, difficulties at work; unsafe neighborhood; racial or religious pressures; natural disasters and loss)
- Additional stressors (loss and grief, uncertainty, exposure to war and terror, political instability, poverty and homelessness).

Past and Present Stressors—What to Ask, Who to Ask, and How

Difficulties in children can have different underlying reasons, and behaviors may serve all manner of functions. Delays and difficulties in ability and behavior may be the primary issue or secondary to other issues in the child's life. The context in which the child lives can help shed light on these functions, along with the attitudes and perceptions toward the child as a whole and the child's 'problems' in particular. When evaluating a child who is showing delays or changes in abilities, it can help to ask and/or note:

- Was the child evaluated before? What for? Were symptoms, behaviors, and issues looked at through a 'big viewfinder' to assess patterns?
- How is the child's development outside of the 'designated complaint'—at school, with peers, with adults, communicatively, academically, physically, emotionally?
- Are issues, behaviors, delays, or problems representing recent changes or were there always difficulties in these areas? If this is an exacerbation, were there changes in the child's life (e.g. at home or at school, recent loss, change in caregiver, medical emergency, or other crises)?
- How is the child's energy level, demeanor, activity level, eating habits, sleep habits? (You might learn of an older child who sleeps in the parents' bed because of nightmares; a grade-school child still using a pacifier.)
- What are the parental dynamics around the child's difficulties and/or issues? Are they on the same page? Do they argue whether the child's issues are real and deserve care or are being blown out of proportion? Does having the child as a 'designated patient' seem to shift attention from or perpetuate other issues?
- Are there other issues/disabilities in the family? Whose? How are those dealt with? Did siblings of either of the parents (or close family members) require therapy by a speech-language pathologist/psychotherapist (depending on the setting)? What for? What was their experience and how did they experience others' attitude toward it?

- If there was/is trauma in the family (directly related to the child or in others in the family), is it discussed? How? Who is it discussed with, how often, and in what context? What does the child understand of it?

The Value of Descriptions

Throughout intake, I ask caregivers to tell me about their child's abilities, personality, things the child enjoys (and whether any have changed recently). Beyond my wish to learn about the child, the ways caregivers describe the child can be very informative (e.g. antsy, lethargic, creative, disinterested, clumsy, manipulative, anxious, lazy, stubborn, graceful, calm). Some provide balanced descriptions of abilities and disabilities, strengths and weaknesses; others do not. When parents list all that is 'wrong with the child' I ask them to tell me 'what is right' and what they find particularly lovable. Some parents are momentarily taken aback, especially if they associated the setting with 'what is wrong,' but gladly fill in other aspects. Others find it difficult to come up with things their child does well or that they find especially lovable. This is important communication about their relationships with the child. It can also point to what the child may not have much experience with (e.g. compliments, being told that he or she is cute, kind, and lovely).

Amy—a professional herself—eloquently described her son's issues with hyperactivity, clumsiness, tantrums, and drooling. She listed all that the six-year-old did not do well, the therapies they'd tried, medication doses, and side effects. When I asked her what she found especially lovable about him, Amy opened and closed her mouth, saying nothing, then broke into tears. "I love him," she said, red with shame. "I mean, I'm his mother. Of course I love him. I'd do anything for him, but there's not much I like about him. Oh, I feel horrible saying this, but his shirt is always wet and he doesn't feel snot on his face and then smears it all over me . . . He breaks everything and bumps into things and sometimes I can't stand him. Nothing is helping to make him like he should be. I hate myself. I don't know what to do anymore . . ."

Amy needed respite. She needed help to manage her issues in relating to her son. Disgust, disappointment, and weariness made it difficult for her to provide him with the warmth and care he deserved, but she was ashamed to ask for help and worried about being judged a bad mother. Speaking about it nonjudgmentally helped clarify something that was likely exacerbating the cycle of rejection and demand. She agreed that addressing her own difficulty would be part of the boy's therapy.

Attachment History—Caregiver Availability and Ability

Shlomy was 3:6 and spoke mostly in short utterances. He was not yet toilet trained, "did not listen well," and threw tantrums when misunderstood. He was 'expelled' from nursery school for biting. Shlomy's behavior worsened after the birth of his sister five months prior. *"Everyone says it is normal sibling rivalry,"* the mother told me during intake. *"I am an only child. I don't know what's normal but I worry for Emma. He is usually sweet with her, but sometimes he gets this look in his eyes, like he really hates her. What if he hurts her? He doesn't know his own strength sometimes."*

Shlomy, cute as a button with cupid lips and cheeks to tempt any grandma's fingers, arrived with his mother for the evaluation well groomed and clearly attentively dressed in slacks and suspenders over a button-down shirt, miniature oxfords, and striped socks. His mother was just as carefully turned out. He regarded me critically from his position by his mother's thigh and did not respond to her coaxing that he take a seat by the small table nearby, clinging to her on the couch instead. I reassured the mother that it was fine for him to take his time, and proceeded to do tantalizing things with magnet pieces at the table. After what Shlomy seemed to judge sufficient time for it to be clear it was his decision and not his mother's, the boy scooted over to the table, eyeing me to ensure he wasn't losing points for 'giving in'. . .

Shlomy's language was indeed delayed. His lexicon was small, his comprehension of concepts limited, and he was behind expectations in many measures of communication. He appeared highly guarded and was conscious of his mother's smallest move. When she needed to use the lavatory (the door within sight of where we sat), he ran after her, insisting on going in with her. This is expected behavior in children his age in a new place, but Shlomy could not bring himself to return to the chair afterward, clinging to his mother, curling in her lap, and stealing side looks at me like an infant who just discovered fear of strangers. His mother was annoyed at his 'refusal to return to work,' and her agitation only seemed to make him clingier. "He is always real clingy," she said to me, a little bitterly.

I spoke with her on the phone later that evening. She apologized for the 'wasted time,' even though I reassured her that this was why my evaluations included more than one session and that anything a child did or did not do was helpful. Children also communicate in how they manage frustration, new situations, difficult feelings, worry, or fatigue. "He wasn't tired," she jumped in, part-defensive, part-accusatory (of the child, it felt). "I let him sleep late. He just got stubborn."

We spoke more about Shlomy's behavior and needs, and I asked again about stresses at home. The mother paused, then shared that she had suffered postpartum depression following his birth. It was mostly her with the baby and she had been unsure what was or was not normal fatigue. She felt embarrassed struggling when she was "supposed to be euphoric" and withdrew from friends, who assumed she had made 'mommy friends.' She didn't. She slept for hours, caring for Shlomy but not really feeling interested in him. Her husband worked long hours and she felt he would not understand. She constantly snapped at him. "It was the hardest six months of my life," she sighed, "until my mom came and saved my life." Reportedly shocked at her daughter's listlessness, she ordered her to the doctor. Antidepressants helped. "It was like a light turned on," Shlomy's mother chocked up. "I could finally breathe. It took time, but it got better and I hired a babysitter for when I wasn't feeling well or Shlomy was too clingy."

I inquired about the recent pregnancy and birth. "I was so worried," Shlomy's mother said. "The doctor monitored me. I had to stop the antidepressants for the pregnancy and it got hard but at least I knew what was happening. As soon as Emma was born, the doctor put me back on the medication and it has been a very different experience." She paused. "I can't get enough of her, and I wonder how much I missed with Shlomy at that age. Those months are a blur."

Postpartum depression may not be disclosed to speech-language pathologists unless it is directly asked about. It's an illness, but parents often feel guilty or ashamed. It is painful to consider and so easier to believe that it had no impact when the child wasn't even speaking. Yet of course it is relevant. Newborns are inherently demanding and rely on caregivers completely for care and interaction. When a caregiver cannot attend to them well enough or consistently enough, babies may find it harder to regulate their bodies, be easily overwhelmed, difficult to soothe, and less able to associate the caregiver with relief and connection (Cozolino 2006, Gaensbauer 2011, Siegel 2012, van der Kolk 2014). Their foundation for relating, communication, self-worth, and understanding of the world can be affected.

Shlomy's mother never intended to harm him. She tried hard to mother him and attended to his physical needs—she fed him and did not leave him in wet diapers—but she struggled to connect with him and was too depressed to truly engage. His presence was a burden, and her guilt and shame fed into her depression. Shlomy's father provided positive connection when he was around, but he traveled a lot for work and was not someone Shlomy could learn to rely on, either. We can wonder: What was it like for Shlomy to not have a besotted caregiver gazing at him, cooing, playing, and interacting with him? What was communicated to him through his mother's disinterest and lethargy? When only his loud cries roused her, what did he understand about the way to get care? It is understandable that he learned to keep near her and keep her engaged, and was desperate for her proximity and responses. The nanny helped—she was warm and loving—and yet what was it like for Shlomy when his mother got depressed again during her second pregnancy? What unnamed memories and fears did her listlessness awaken in his toddler understanding? How was it for him to see his mother interact with the new infant in ways he—even without knowing how to explain it—had to have yearned for?

Young children have limited language skills and therefore often communicate by behavior and affect. Toddlers commonly display distress in biting or hitting, tantrums, clinginess, and overcontrolling whatever they can (e.g. food, toileting). It is effective communication that can backfire. The very ways Shlomy controlled connection—crying, clinging, refusing to toilet-train—irritated and overwhelmed his mother, recreating dismissal and rejection that made him even more anxious and her more reactive. Both mother and son were replaying attachment conflict through anxiety, shame, and guilt.

Discussing attachment behaviors as communications was not about blame or explaining away a language delay, but about understanding what contributed to Shlomy's communication profile and coping. It was an important part of assessing his skills and planning an optimal intervention, because it also offered hope for how to help support his availability for learning. Shlomy's mother agreed that she deserved help to process what had been a very difficult time for her, and accepted my recommendation that she seek counseling. Therapy helped her manage guilt and shame and provided her with tools for managing her own feelings and for containing Shlomy's difficult feelings so he could regulate better. Their improved connection eased the anxiety between them, and her sensitivity assuaged the jealousy Shlomy felt (and expressed) toward his infant sister. Everyone's communication got better. In Shlomy's family—as in many others—attending to attachment issues (in this case through parent counseling alongside speech therapy for the child) improved the effectiveness of intervention. It calmed hypervigilance and stress all around and increased Shlomy's availability for language learning, processing, and use (more about clinical collaboration in Chapter 16).

It is often helpful to understand what took place during early communication and attachment. This does not mean that attachment must be perfect, just 'good enough' (to borrow Winnicott's term). Not every disruption in attachment will or should affect development and behavior, but it is worth asking about attachment and early communication patterns during assessments. If nothing else, the history of caregiver availability and abilities can shed light on the relational environment the child grew up in and the 'messages' he or she may have internalized. Some helpful things to consider inquiring about:

- Attachment difficulties following birth (NICU, separation from the baby, difficult recovery from C-section, medications that made it hard to care for the baby)
- Postpartum depression
- Loss in the family (loss of a sibling of the child or parent? How and what effect did it have on connection with/worry for this child?)
- Caregiving history (Who is the main caregiver? Were they ever unavailable? Why? At what age, for how long? Who cared for the baby? Other caregiver changes?)
- Caretaking beliefs and habits (e.g. sleep and eating habits/schedule; response to crying; use of pacifier/blanket/suckling; family bed or crib; conflicts between caregivers about the 'right way' to child-care?)
- Caregivers' language and fluency (What language/s did caregivers speak with the child? How well did they speak them?—when caregivers are instructed

or feel compelled to use a language they are not proficient in and/or are self-conscious using, it can affect connection and communication.)

Fostering, Adoption, Loss, and Divorce

Foster-Care

A child in foster-care is a child at high risk for trauma history. Whatever the cause for removal from parental care—abuse, neglect, violence, loss of parent, incarceration of a parent—the separation itself is a significant stressor for any child, let alone the circumstances leading to and following it. Shifts in foster-care placement and failed reunification can increase attachment disruption, loss, and uncertainty. They can impact a child's occupation with safety and stability at the cost of availability for development, exploration, communication, and learning.

Whenever a child is in foster-care or has a history of foster-care placement, it can be helpful to ask:

- When was the child placed in foster-care? (how long ago)
- How old was the child when first placed in foster-care?
- What was the reason for fostering? (abuse/neglect, violence, parental illness, loss of parent, parental incarceration, etc.)
- Who was the child placed with? (family fostering? general fostering?)
- How many placements did the child have (during what period of time), including reunifications if there were any, and/or emergency fostering placement/s?
- Was there a change in language? (e.g. Spanish at home, English in foster-care)
- Are there visitations with the biological parent? How and where do they take place? How does the child do before/during/after them?
- Are there siblings and does the child live with them?
- Is there an extended family? What is the child's connection with them? Do they express conflict about the custody loss? Is there disbelief/blame toward the child?
- Is/was the child receiving counseling?
- Did someone follow the child's development throughout? Does anyone know the child's whole history?

Access to history in foster-children varies considerably. Sometimes much is documented, while at other times information is sketchy, and current caregivers (foster-parents, biological parent after reunification, or adoptive parent) have only skeletal data of the child's shuttling through the system and loss of custody. Information about developmental milestones, medical history, interventions, therapies, and issues may be patchy and make it hard to get a good sense of the child's development. When that happens, the fractured history of itself provides a mirror to the experience of the child: lack of continuity, instability, confusion, and unpredictability. It is not surprising that a child whose own life narrative is fraught with 'holes' and ruptures could have difficulty narrating experiences, connecting causation, or understanding sequence.

Adoption

Unless it takes place immediately after birth, adoption implies a history of disrupted attachment and loss. Adoption also increases the risk that there was prenatal exposure to stress through maternal stress, intrauterine exposure to alcohol and other substances, malnutrition in the mother, and mental health issues in the mother (Albers et al 2005, Miller 2005, Yehuda et al 2005). Prenatal and early history may not be known when children were abandoned to orphanages or adopted from other countries. However, available information can still be of help:

- How old was the child at adoption?
- What is known of the child's prenatal development and circumstances? Is the mother known? Was she well/well nourished? Any indications the child was exposed to substances?
- How did the child become eligible for adoption? (foster-care, orphanage, abandonment, prearranged adoption, or surrogacy?)
- What language/s was the child exposed to before adoption? Since?
- What kind of care did the child receive pre-adoption? (e.g. biological family, foster-family, or institution? What were the conditions? Did caregivers change a lot?)
- Were there medical/developmental issues?
- Did the child receive therapies? What for, which ones, by whom?
- Were there siblings/peers the child was close to? Where are they? (Did they remain in the orphanage/get adopted elsewhere/return to the parent?)
- Did the child suffer any other loss? (e.g. pet, grandparent)

Loss

Death is a natural part of the life cycle. Not all loss is traumatic or results in ongoing grief that distracts a child from attending and developing. However, children can suffer significant loss, and their understanding of grief can be complicated by their comprehension of what happened and what it means (Nader & Salloum 2011). Beyond the effect of young age on perception and beliefs, the presence of language issues increases the risk for misconception and confusion. It is important to ask about loss. Adults may not always know what losses are most meaningful to a particular child, and children can experience grief for losses adults are not aware were so profound. Caregivers usually mention a loss of a parent or sibling, but other losses (e.g. loss of a relative the child was close to, a friend, a beloved pet) may not be shared unless asked about. If parents do not bring up the loss of a child, it may be because it is too painful and they cannot see the relevance to another child's communication. However, what they do or do not speak of can mirror the family's way of communicating around loss, grief, and hardship—beliefs that can become interwoven with the child's understanding of reality and communication.

Ken's preschool teacher voiced concerns about his listening comprehension and vocabulary and wondered whether the 4:6-year-old had a language delay. When his parents called me for an evaluation, they shared that Ken's paternal grandmother, whom he saw a few times a year and who adored him, passed away quite unexpectedly two months prior. Ken was deemed too young to attend the wake or funeral and the loss did not seem to occupy him beyond stating empathically in the days following the death that "Daddy is sad because Gramma died." Ken's mother noted in passing that "maybe Doc's death a few months before that helped Ken understand Granma's death."

Doc was the family's dog. When Ken was born, Doc saw the newborn as an extension of his pack and literally guarded the baby's crib and then toddler-bed each night till morning. The week Ken turned four years old, Doc was taken to the vet and diagnosed with advanced cancer that was causing the dog extreme suffering. Ken's parents let the vet put him down. As a way of explaining the dog's disappearance without worrying Ken with pain and cancer, Ken's parents told him that Doc had to go to the vet and that the vet "had to put him to sleep." The boy reportedly accepted this placidly enough, and when he periodically asked his parents about the dog over the next few days, they patiently repeated what they'd said before, believing that he "needed to hear what he already knew."

Doc's death coincided with Ken's beginning preschool. When a few weeks later the child became clingy and fussy in the evenings and woke repeatedly at night, the parents were advised that he was "adjusting" and "overtired" with the long school days and that nightmares were normal at his age. Ken rarely mentioned Doc, but his parents believed he 'channeled' his love of dogs into having almost everything in his room have a dog motif. They found it adorable.

Knowing about Doc's death proved very helpful. It explained the child's dramatic reaction to a common story he chose for me to read during the evaluation: "Harry the Dirty Dog." Ken seemed anxious and sad, but when I asked him if he wanted us to read a different story, he shook his head 'no.' His mother chuckled mirthlessly and noted that "he is obsessive about dog stories" and cried if they did not read the "dog stories first."

Alert to the contradiction between his reported enthusiasm and sadness, I asked Ken if he liked dogs. He nodded but then shook his head, "only Doc."

"Only Doc?" the mother stated, surprised, "Everything in your bedroom is 'dog'— your bedspread, stuffed animals, books, puzzles—you keep asking for dog things. I thought you loved dogs!"

"Only Doc," he repeated.

"How come?" I asked gently.

He hung big eyes on me, then looked down at the open book in front of us and gently traced the illustration of the black and white dog. Harry of the story was very different than the large brown mutt Doc had been, and the tenderness of the boy's touch belied his declaration.

"It looks like you like this dog too, a little bit," I prompted.

Ken shrugged, paused. "Maybe he goes to the vet," he murmured.

"Hmm. . ." I wasn't sure where he was going with this but wanted to see if he'd say more.

He looked up at me, eyes brimming. "Maybe he goes to the vet, he can wake up Doc."

Ken has been accumulating dogs in a search for one that may know the vet Doc had gone to, so that they can wake Doc up from the sleep the vet 'put' him into and remind him to come home. Sleep became confusing for Ken. He did not like being put to bed because it made him miss his dog even more. It reminded him that sleep took his beloved dog away. He was scared to have his parents asleep, so he cried to wake them up to reassure himself that they could wake, unlike Doc, who slept and slept and slept . . . Ken could not understand why no one was waking Doc. His parents seemed sad that Doc was sleeping and still they did not go to the vet to wake him and bring him home. When he asked where Doc was, they just kept saying he was 'put to sleep.' Ken had to go to sleep at night, too. What if he did not wake up? Or his parents—how long would they sleep for? What if he misses them and they do not wake up?

For Ken, the death of his grandmother was sad only because it saddened his father. His parents used the word "dead" and he understood it meant Grandma not coming to visit anymore. She had never been part of his everyday, and her death was abstract and quite separate from the loss of Doc. Ken's parents did not realize it. To them being 'put to sleep' was synonymous with 'dead' and so they thought Ken understood that Doc was dead just like his grandmother and would not return. It was not synonymous to Ken, who did not understand how being put to sleep could sometimes mean being gone for a very long time. He missed Doc terribly, but no one else seemed to be waiting. So Ken looked for Doc in every dog he saw, in every picture-book with dogs. Maybe if he found a dog who could find Doc, that dog would help wake him. Dogs became both trigger and compulsion. Learning about this loss and how it affected Ken was important for his evaluation and treatment planning. Doc's loss had become the focal point of Ken's attention and he had little energy left for things like listening and exploration.

Divorce

Asking about divorce can be a legal necessity (e.g. who should grant permission for releasing information to school or other clinicians, who is allowed to bring the child to therapy or pick her up) and important logistically (who pays for therapy, who comes with the child, who should be notified of a cancellation or arrange rescheduling). It can also be clinically relevant with regard to its impact on the child: What was the divorce like and on what grounds, what was life like at home before the separation, during, since? How long did the process take? How did it affect the child's life in matters daily and relational—did they need to move schools, move homes, leave behind friends, separate from siblings? How often do they see the other parent? How is it for them? What do they understand about the reason and meaning of the divorce? How much animosity is there between the parents? Is the child the mouthpiece for interparent communication? Does the child (have to) take sides?

Divorce always includes some measure of loss and is a significant event in children's lives, representing a time of strain and change. That said, not all divorce is traumatic or developmentally disruptive. Sometimes divorce brings stability and reduced stress, and many parents put the children first and co-parent effectively and kindly. Children can adapt well to split households, step-siblings, half-siblings and step-parents, 'gaining' more caregivers who love and attend to them in the bargain. Children can learn that change does not need to mean that all is lost or love destroyed.

In other families, divorce can become a devastating wrenching with continued conflict that can weave chronic stress into both everyday and special occasions (e.g. who comes to birthdays, where they'd be for holidays). Children may feel they have no voice beyond the one they are made to parrot for this or the other parent and that their needs are not heard or matter. Giving them a voice may begin with learning more about the circumstances that may have silenced it.

"It Is Like She Just Checks Out Completely"—Listening to What Is Said—The Power of Others' Observations

Assessments can be filled with test items, checklists, rating scales, and questionnaires. In the flurry of data, it is important to listen to the wording and manner of responses, especially for supposedly 'offhanded' phrases or descriptors. Assessments that continue into 'diagnostic treatment' often spread beyond the bounds of first sessions and allow more input. On some level, every session is a continuation of assessment. Whether we see a child for an evaluation only or for long-term treatment, the child, caregivers, siblings, educators, along with medical and clinical personnel, often fill in things that no checklist can.

Nelly, the seven-year-old daughter of a physician and a financier, was diagnosed by an educational psychologist to have a language learning disorder NOS (not otherwise specified) and 'atypical ADHD.' It was recommended she get speech-language therapy and attend "behavior skills group" (to improve attending and reduce the 'silent-treatment tantrums' of the child refusing to respond). Nelly's history included occupational therapy as a toddler for what the parents described as 'sensory issues' (refusing socks, not tolerating seams on clothing, etc.). "She graduated out of it," the father noted, "but I still think she's oversensitive." The mother added that Nelly was very picky—where they go for brunch, which stores and for how long—and that the psychologist suggested it was about control. Classroom teachers, too, described Nelly as "unreasonably stubborn." "Maybe it is manipulation," Nelly's mother sighed, "but sometimes I don't know. She doesn't argue much or try to get your attention. It is like she just checks out completely."

Nelly was a well-cared-for child with two attentive and involved parents who tried to do the best for her. There were no major traumas or losses in her life, yet her parents' wording had me wonder whether she was overwhelmed. I recommended an updated assessment by an occupational therapist, which showed that Nelly was still very hypersensitive, that normal-range sensations exceeded her tolerance, but that she had learned to go numb. Numbing helped her manage but also meant she did not learn to desensitize or regulate, remaining hypersensitive and anxious of stimuli. She also had hyperacusis—oversensitive hearing—sounds that others found reasonable hurt her ears. It was the reason Nelly had refused certain restaurants or stores—the reverberation, loud music, or other noises put her teeth on edge. She could not understand how others seemed to not care or even enjoy what she found painful. The only thing she could do was to shut down, sometimes preemptively. When her parents (grudgingly) remained at home or changed a restaurant, it reinforced the effectiveness of this coping but avoided the issue.

Nelly returned to occupational therapy and began therapy with me. Her oversensitivity was much improved by desensitization, and some modifications helped reduce her overwhelm (e.g. a personal FM system at school, noise-canceling headphones in noisy places). She learned to communicate saturation verbally before reaching "the too-much-point" and to identify what about a place/event was difficult. Preplanning (e.g. alternating noisy places with quiet ones) and establishing an 'I-need-out' signal with her parents and teachers also helped. No longer missing interaction or instruction to numbing or to stress, Nelly closed gaps quickly and her attention issues resolved.

Other examples of worth-listening-to wordings:

- "He is crying like he's really hurting"—the parent of a cranky and language-delayed toddler who could only be soothed when held, sometimes whole nights. Reflux was ruled out and the pediatrician suggested it was best to "let him cry a bit" so he could get used to sleeping in his bed, but the parents "could not bear his crying." Further testing showed food sensitivities that caused congestion, and inflammation that hurt his head when it was not elevated.
- "She did not sleep through the night for months afterwards. We were all barely awake through that time"—the mother of a child with a learning delay whose younger brother got hurt in a scalding accident.

- "Oh, he was never very loving . . . It makes everything harder, you know"—a mother about the boy she adopted at three from foster-care.
- "He makes such strange mistakes, it's almost like the words get scrambled in his head"—a teacher about a student in her class. He was found to have auditory processing issues.

Taking Note of Your Own Reactions—the Informative Power of Yawning, and Other Sneaky Signs

It is an important clinical tool to be aware of our thoughts, reactions, sensations, and feelings when we are with clients (Figley 1995, Fonagy & Target 1997, Gomez 2012, Howell 2011, Wallin 2007). This is especially valuable when our reactions feel out-of-synch or unexplained—we may be picking up on 'something in the room.' Clients and caregivers bring unexpressed issues into the interaction, which get communicated in unexpected reactions in the clinician. The unspoken is especially important to be aware of when dealing with traumatized children, who may not know how to verbalize their experiences, may have needed to adopt more than one way of being, or learned to numb or hide their emotions to survive (Silberg 1998, 2013, Waters 2005, Wieland 2011).

Just like clients, clinicians have histories and needs, blind spots and tender buttons. Clients may touch us deeply, infuriate us, and remind of others loved or hated. Their actions (and inactions) can frustrate or inspire. While subjectivity certainly complicates clinical objectivity, it is also the richness of connection that provides therapeutic interactions with healing potential (Cozolino 2014, Howell 2011, Wallin 2007, van der Kolk 2014). Nowhere is this truer than when treating communication and trauma issues, which can isolate and deprive of connection. Whether in assessment or in the continued reassessing of therapy, clinical attunement allows us to identify what gets evoked in us, the information it carries about the interaction, and what in the client's needs (or our own) is awakened.

Feelings 'leak.' We pick up on clients' feelings and they will pick up on ours. In fact, we expect clients to feel the authenticity of our praise, caring, empathy, pride. Other feelings can get communicated, too. A quarter-century of clinical experience (and personal life along the way) taught me to notice rather than judge: When I have a strong reaction to a child (or parent), I wonder if it communicates unmet needs (in me or the other) and what these may be about. For example, children's behavior very rarely irritates or disappoints me, so if such feelings ever rise in me, I reflect about what could be irritating or disappointing: Are there things I should be doing and am not? Am I asking too much too soon? Is the child irritated or disappointed and I have missed or misinterpreted it? What have I not understood? Similarly, when a parent evokes impatience or frustration in me, I wonder what has not been said: What do they need that I am not 'getting'? What makes it hard to openly acknowledge? What do I need and did not attend to?

Yawning, fatigue, headache, rumbling tummies, wandering thoughts, irritation and restlessness, spacing out, nodding off: These are important communicators. They can tell us we are not doing enough to take care of ourselves, or of old triggered dynamics we are at risk of (or are) replaying. They may also reflect unspoken issues with a client. Either way, our own bodies can become effective sound-chambers for the unsaid.

Every child and every assessment is different, yet all interactions are ongoing processes where knowledge layers to fill in what we know about the children, how they learn, their attitudes and those others hold about them, their history and reactions to it, the skills they acquired and how they do (or do not) use them. The same is true about awareness of the possibility of trauma and developmental impact. Good history, an eye out for stressors and the supports the child had (or did not have) for managing them, the child's attachment history and losses, what is and is not said, our own feelings and reactions: All have a role in 'hearing' the communications of children who come to us for voice and help.

Part 5

Mending Meaning

Intervention Strategies, Collaboration,
and the Importance of Taking Care

14 Psychoeducation and Everyday Tools for Reducing Overwhelm

Traumatized children can be challenging. Their behaviors can seem erratic, uncaring, deceitful, and confusing. Inconsistencies can make it difficult to ascertain their abilities and skills (Ford & Courtois 2013, Heineman 1998, Heller & Lapierre 2012, Kagan 2004, Pearce & Pezzot-Pearce 1997, Putnam 1997, Silberg 1998, 2013, Smith et al 1998, Waters 2005, Wieland 2011, Yehuda 2005, 2011). Parents, teachers, caretakers, educators, pediatricians, nurses, coaches, dentists, and other child professionals can benefit from recognizing and understanding children's reactions, and need practical tools for effective response. Children with developmental, relational, educational, and emotional difficulties are at high risk for trauma and overwhelm (Benedict et al 1990, Crosse et al 1993, Goldson 1998, Knutson & Sullivan 1993, Sullivan & Knutson 1998, 2000, Sullivan et al 1987, 2009). Realizing why children present a certain way, what triggers them, and how to minimize distress can improve communication and connection for everyone involved.

Advocating for Trauma-Sensitive Assessment and Therapy

Children end up at clinics and offices for all manner of reasons. Those who fall behind, forget directions, or do not express themselves well often get sent to speech-language pathologists. Those with misbehaviors, school refusal, or anxieties are taken to psychologists. Children who seem unable to tolerate stimuli may see an occupational therapist; children in pain, physicians and physical therapists, etc. Awareness to trauma and communication is important in all cases. Speech-language pathologists should watch for risk factors and clues in history and clinical presentation that may indicate need for trauma assessment by a psychotherapist. Psychotherapists need to keep aware of the prevalence and manifestation of language and communication issues in children with trauma histories and whether assessment by a speech-language pathologist is indicated. All clinicians can guide caregivers in minimizing and attending to overwhelm.

In a perfect world, every child will have access to sensitive care that minimizes overwhelm, and receive informed care if trauma does happen. We are not there yet. Limited awareness of traumatic impact on children's communication and learning means that many children who struggle do not get assessed for trauma (Waters 2005). Cuts to funding often prioritize trauma referrals to blatant abuse cases or short-term advice after a tragedy or disaster. There remains a troubling tendency to minimize the prevalence and impact of trauma on children (Silberg 2013, Waters 2005, Wieland 2011), due to misinformation, politics, denial, taboos, and conflicts of interest (Freyd & Birrell 2013).

Nonetheless many professionals and caregivers are increasingly aware of the ramifications of trauma, the long-term impact of untreated overwhelm, and the availability of effective remedies (Gomez 2012, Kluft 1985, Levine & Kline 2007, Perry & Szalavitz 2006, Silberg 1998, 2013, Waters 2005, Wieland 2011, Yehuda 2005, 2011). Multidisciplinary research into developmental trauma is already serving to inform professionals and the public (Cozolino 2006, 2014, Gaensbauer 2011, Scaer 2014, Schore 2012, Siegel 2012, van der Kolk 2014). Together we can help increase the numbers of trauma-informed lawmakers, educators, and clinicians who understand the implications of trauma and can offer children much needed support.

Reframing Problem Behaviors

Most people accept that bad things happen to children. However, knowing about children's difficult beginnings does not always translate into understanding why they don't listen in school, behave inappropriately, or 'act oppositional' (Silberg 2013, Smith et al 1998, Waters 2005, Wieland 2011, Yehuda 2005, 2011). Many of the coping behaviors of traumatized children can be disruptive, problematic, and unacceptable. Spitting, pushing, cursing, giving lip, throwing tantrums (or chairs . . .), ignoring, denying, and lying are rarely endearing. Teachers and caregivers can find "challenging kids" difficult to connect with, and because post-traumatic reactions can be out of awareness and/or control, misunderstandings and additional acting out often follow. By placing a difficult child's behavior in the context of traumatic overwhelm, adults are more likely to hold a caring and rewarding connection. For both child and adult, understanding fosters better attachment and regulation.

Jennifer's teachers saw her as "promiscuous" and "disgusting." The eight-year-old constantly had "her hands down her pants," displayed "seductive" behaviors, and used "gutter language." She was almost universally disliked and often in detention for "misbehavior" (and her discomfiting presence). The gym teacher was especially uncomfortable and worried the child could get him in trouble if people misinterpreted her behaviors as his fault. He preferred to exclude Jennifer from his class for "bad influence" and "inappropriateness." Already struggling academically, Jennifer kept missing instruction. She was also frustrated, lonely, and locked in impossible binds of hunger for connection, inability to verbalize her needs, and punishment when she attempted to get them met.

Staff knew that Jennifer had been molested as a preschooler and was in foster-care because of parental maltreatment. Both parents had addictions. The father admitted to "fooling around" with Jennifer and the mother reportedly let her drug dealer "spend time" with the small girl. Teachers rationally understood where Jennifer "learned this stuff" but they still judged her ongoing sexualized behaviors as somehow complicit. "She seems so into it," the classroom teacher grumbled. "Like this is what she wants."

I met with the teachers to discuss the realities of entrapment and the desperate need of young children to make meaning and adapt to whatever circumstances maltreating adults place them in. Jennifer's undesirable behaviors were the product of the reality she had lived. She communicated with adults the way adults showed her to—sexually. Like many sexually abused children, Jennifer may have learned to initiate sexual contact to control anxiety about when she might be abused. It was also possible that sexual contact was the only way Jennifer received warmth or contact. She might have learned to associate attention with sexual advances and receiving comfort with sexual stimulation. Jennifer was 'telling' her reality through her behavior and it was up to us to understand and reframe her needs in healthier ways, not to push her away for internalizing realities she endured.

Reframing helped. "I knew Jennifer had sexual abuse," the gym teacher admitted, "but I didn't really think what it had to be like. Makes me mad—a small child stuck with adults doing these things." Another teacher nodded: "Maybe that's how she knows to get through life. Breaks your heart, it does." With the child's behaviors in context, the teachers found more compassion toward her and became less shaming. They were also more open to noticing and reinforcing instances of good behavior, something Jennifer was hungry for and responded very favorably to. With increased positive attention for nonsexualized things, Jennifer seemed to have 'less need' for inappropriate behavior. Her teachers also became protective of her. When a paraprofessional commented, "This girl behaves like a ho'," the classroom teacher jumped in with "This is what her lousy-excuse-for-parents taught her! Not her fault. The shame's on them that did not protect her!"

Clarifying Boundaries and Expectations

Understanding and reframing children's behaviors certainly helps increase compassion and empathy and lowers frustration. However, understanding and reframing are not enough. It is also important to have safe boundaries and realistic expectations that are clearly stated and that the child understands and can succeed in keeping. For traumatized children, this is no easy feat. Children learn about boundaries and how they are kept (or breached) through experiences with implicit and explicit modeling of boundaries with them. Traumatized children often had boundaries (of their bodies, safety, and tolerance) violated or ignored (Diseth 2006, Gaensbauer 2011, Silberg 2013, Wieland 2011, van der Kolk 2014). They may not know how to recognize, keep, or request boundaries. They can stand too close, ignore cues for avoiding or stopping touch, miss signs of discomfort, and misinterpret approval or denial. They may hit, grab, push, pull, lean into, rub against, take, hide, deny. They often do not know how to explain why.

"You would think he'd know how it feels to be hit," Jimmy's foster-mother complained, *"after all the fists he got at his bio home, he should be the last person to hit others..."*

"Or," I offered, *"he is hitting because it is how he saw frustration expressed and power displayed. It may even be the only way he knows to show he cares."*

"A very strange show of care—knocking someone's teeth out," Jimmy's foster-mother muttered, politely dismissing my interpretation. She was speaking literally: She'd rushed another foster-child to the dentist after Jimmy (age nine) boxed him in the teeth, loosening a brand new incisor.

"Yes," I repeated meaningfully, *"strange way indeed to show care..."*

She paused and took a breath. *"I forgot."*

Jimmy was removed to foster-care at five years old, after his mother's boyfriend 'disciplined' him by punching him in the face and knocking out two teeth. Jimmy's mature teeth have grown in since, along with his use of violence on others...

Understanding Jimmy's behavior did not mean he could continue smashing people's teeth out when he got frustrated or felt the need to 'discipline' someone. Like other children whose bodies were exploited, intruded upon, disrespected, or neglected, he needed opportunities to learn and practice boundaries. He needed to be able to make mistakes, get gentle correction, and be praised when he succeeded. We cannot assume traumatized children know how to keep body boundaries or other boundaries. In fact, we should assume they don't.

Body Boundaries

Body boundaries are often taught to children in reference to "good touch, bad touch" as part of sexual abuse prevention. More generally these include people's right to their bodies and the right to say "no" to what is unacceptable—sexual or not—without apology or guilt. Under normal conditions, children should have the power to stop any contact they find uncomfortable or unwelcome. They should be able to have it stopped first and explain why later, or even not explain at all beyond "I don't like this" or "I don't want to."

Things get tricky when conditions are not normal, such as if a child needs to be restrained for his safety or get medical treatment he does not approve of. It can be even more confusing when treatment involves intimate parts that children were taught were "no touch" areas or when their demand to "not touch there" or "let me go" cannot be followed. Because stress reduces language processing (van der Kolk 2014), children may find it difficult to process explanations for why rules are breached, and their confusion can increase. Even in the context of overall respect, boundaries can become untrustworthy after a breach, let alone for children whose boundaries were not kept and who have no blueprint of having power over their bodies.

Anytime a child's boundaries have been violated—even for reasons adults believe were justified—it is important to repair them afterward. To explain what happened, validate the 'rules' and how and why this deviated from them, acknowledge the child's rage and fear, apologize for breaking promises, and reaffirm how boundaries are still real and important. Depending on the child's distress, distrust, and confusion, it might mean repeating the repair several times and providing opportunities for the child to 'test' that the rules indeed matter. Without repair, children may worry not only about the rule that broke but that all rules are unreliable.

Careful teaching and explanation is even more essential to children who suffered ongoing trauma and disrespect of their boundaries (Silberg 2013). Children cannot be expected to 'maintain good boundaries' without having had a way to internalize and establish what those are or why to keep them. We cannot assume that children understand boundaries by watching how they treat others, either. Some children learned to respect other people's boundaries (or risk serious harm, abandonment, rejection, etc.) but do not extend these to themselves. Their needs remain unmet by people mistaking their lack of limiting for 'not minding,' and it leaves the children vulnerable for continued victimization.

It goes without saying that anyone working with traumatized children should be acutely aware of boundaries and of the children's possible difficulty with understanding or verbalizing them. If a caregiver must restrain a child to prevent her from harming herself or others, these interventions must be followed with verbalizing the breach of boundary, apologizing for it, and ensuring that everyday boundaries and their limits are explained. The same goes for the child's behavior toward others: We cannot assume children know or understand.

Using Touch with Traumatized Children

The daily care and protection of young (or disabled) children often requires physical contact: donning and doffing coats and mittens, zipping zippers, crossing safely, wiping noses, washing up. There are also therapeutic needs like working hand-over-hand, correcting posture, and offering comfort and support. Maintaining good boundaries around children should not mean refraining from affectionate or supportive touch. Touch itself is not the problem but how and why it is provided. Touching should always be done with care and respect, never in anger, and with the child's level of comfort or discomfort in mind. Children may not verbalize their comfort with proximity but they communicate it in their bodies. They may express dilemmas by simultaneously leaning into and away, getting close and retreating.

In my practice, unless I need to keep a child safe (e.g. from falling), I usually wait for the child to initiate contact. How and when he or she does so
tells me a lot. Some high-risk kids watch my interaction with others before
they attempt proximity. Others reach out to me right away, though this does
not necessarily indicate comfort with closeness—a child may be testing to see
what I would do.

Most children allow and even seek touch once they feel they have the right
to refuse it, stop it, and move away from it. However, for children whose body
boundaries have been compromised, even the gentlest touch may not be comforting. Sexually abused children can find affection scary and triggering, not
knowing 'where it leads' or what is expected. Oversensitive children can find
even casual touch intolerable. Neglected children may be confused by affection,
and physically abused children may not know how to interpret touch that is
not aggressive. Children's own behaviors often reinforce unpleasant contact. If
restrained, grabbed, and tugged back, they may fight back, reinforcing cycles of
aggression. They might shut down and 'leave' their bodies, reinforcing dissociation. Touch communicates, and traumatized children may need to be taught a
'vocabulary' of tolerable and safe physical connection.

Teaching boundaries includes narrating what they can expect from others:
what will and will not happen. This can put in words what was left unspoken,
and help form a baseline for verbalizing 'body language,' needs, and reactions.
Erring on the side of overexplaining, I tell children I will never do anything
intentionally to hurt them. I ask that if by mistake I do anything uncomfortable,
they let me know so I can stop and apologize. For some children this is novelty:
They never had control over adults' actions in relation to their bodies, let alone
permission to tell adults they did wrong and have adults apologize. I explain that
unless it is an emergency where I must keep them safe, they can always stop me
or move away.

Then we practice. They give me a hand and pull it out, get close and move
away. If my work involves touching their face for oral-motor and articulation
work, we practice my touching their cheek or lips and their saying "stop" or "no,"
where I immediately do so. For reciprocity and mirroring I often have children
do on me the exercises I do with them. And so we practice my saying "no" and
"stop," so they can get praise for good listening. It provides experience with being
the one who stops an action and chooses to respect another's body, and helps
children regulate their touch, improving mastery over their bodies near other
people. We discuss (and practice) how people differ in what feels okay and the
body clues that show that someone is uncomfortable. We practice how to ask
permission and how to apologize if a breach occurred.

When children are aggressive, I verbalize it and remind them of rules we have
already established. I might say, "Please stop this hitting/pinching/poking. It
hurts." If they continue, I might hold them back gently and explain: "You are

hurting me. Please stop. I am holding your arms so you won't punch anymore. Punching is not okay. It hurts. I don't want you to hurt me and I don't want you to get hurt. I see you're upset. Let's talk about what is making you upset." When children stop hitting, I ask if I can let them go without their hitting, and then apologize for holding them and repeat why I had done so. We talk about what happened, what they felt, how they feel now. If they hit another child, I would ask them to apologize to the child so that both children can be assured that physical aggression demands an apology. However, I rarely if ever demand an apology for hitting me—children usually offer it themselves when I model my regret over having to restrain them.

When children touch me inappropriately—and some do—I adjust their position and calmly explain my own boundaries (e.g. "I am moving your hand because it is touching my breasts and my breasts are private parts of my body. You can still sit next to me and you can hold my hand or touch my arm instead," or "This kind of touching is not comfortable for me, but you are welcome to lean into me/hug me this way instead . . ."). I use language the children understand and verbalize both the reason for the changed position and the fact that they are still welcome to maintain proximity. I stay matter-of-fact and non-shaming, and I never push children away or punish them for touching me that way: They are being as appropriate as they know to be according to the rules they understand. It is up to me (and all adults) to recognize their underlying needs and provide them with alternative rules that work better.

I don't necessarily touch every child I work with, but to me touch is an integral part of communication and understanding of boundaries, especially with young children, those with developmental delays, and/or those who experienced distorted interrelating. Touch is in fact part of many therapeutic interactions and can be used well with care and awareness. That said, not everyone shares the same level of comfort with proximity. If you are uncomfortable with touch, you should probably not use it. Ambivalence about physical contact is always communicated. Children—especially maltreated children—can be acutely perceptive of such ambivalences and will likely interpret it as shaming.

More Boundaries

In the complex strata of interpersonal boundaries, children need modeling for acceptable words and actions that can allow them to express themselves without damaging property, people, or relationships. They need to learn how to express difficult feelings such as frustration, rejection, fear, rage, shame, worry, as well as exuberance, excitement, joy, and affection. Here, too, practice is essential. Children need direction and opportunities to practice acceptable behavior in neutral situations before they can be expected to use it when flooded with a feeling. It takes more than "we don't do that" or "hitting is not okay" to learn how to express anger without aggression. Children need clear steps toward goals they can attain. Setting a bar too high sets them up for failure, frustration, and more shame, while successes help children learn how it feels to regulate actions and keep a boundary, and how it feels to be praised and experience pride.

Some children learn boundaries quickly. Others need many repetitions, tiny increments, and multiple reminders. For children to manage maintaining boundaries while emotional, they need to be able to self-regulate, perceive and process a situation, and come up with an appropriate reaction for the time, place, and person—a complex goal that ties in to many other skills children may need help with. One way to increase a child's ability to apply boundaries is to anticipate tricky situations and review boundaries beforehand. For example, I may remind children of the need to stay patient and keep their bodies calm during an upcoming wait in the lunchroom. I may review how they can do so: be aware of their bodies, their distance from others, where their hands are, things they can say or do if someone crowds them. Later we discuss what worked, what did not, and why. Placing experiences and actions into context helps behaviors become more conscious, better processed, and ultimately better controlled.

Teaching and Modeling the 'Tool-Kit'

Reframing behaviors and teaching boundaries form a good baseline for connection, but traumatized children can still get triggered by trauma reminders. When that happens, they might react from overwhelm, fight/flight, or numbing, unable to apply new behaviors. To help them get grounded, caregivers, educators, and clinicians need concrete ways that work. Some children find it helpful to be reminded to take a few deep breaths. Deep breathing helps lower the neurological arousal that takes place during a stress reaction (Levine & Kline 2007, van der Kolk 2014). It is important to practice such deep breathing when children are calm, so that their bodies can more easily remember how to do so when upset.

Other children find prearranged hand movements (e.g. lowering the palm in a gentle 'calm down' motion) helpful in calming them enough to listen and orient to their surroundings (Yehuda 2011). Education professionals often use hand motions and may be comfortable with using them relatively unobtrusively in classroom settings. These motions, too, need to be practiced when the child is calm. Practice augments understanding and reinforces the calm-down association so that it is familiar and established if the child gets triggered.

Excerpt from "Leroy—It Is Almost like He Is Two Children" (Yehuda in Wieland 2011).

. . . I practice it (the hand motion) with Leroy in our session. I explain to him what it means and how it can remind him to calm down even when his mind is too busy to listen. I have one of the stuffed animals "get really angry" and then prompt it to calm down and "it does." It is then Leroy's turn to "calm" a series of toys having

tantrums and—best of all—to "help me calm down" when I pretend to get really upset. He loves the new "game."

When I ask him, as review, what the hand motion helps him do, he pauses for a moment, then says, "It make it more better in my head and I see you."

The Tool-Kit

Sometimes children need more than a reminder to take a deep breath, or a hand motion to get grounded and reorient to the 'here and now.' Years of working with traumatized children and with their caregivers helped identify several steps that can be particularly helpful. These were developed into a 'tool-kit' which has since been taught and implemented internationally (ISSTD Child & Adolescent Committee 2009, Yehuda 2011). The tool-kit can be utilized by educators, caregivers, clinicians, or other adults working with a child, at any time a child is in distress, whether one knows what the trigger was or not. The sequential steps can appear long, but in actuality take very little time and can be implemented unobtrusively. As associations form between the first step and subsequent calming, children often get grounded even more quickly.

1. *Grounding.* This helps a child reorient to the present. As soon as you notice the child beginning to dissociate, approach gently and let the child know where he is and who he is—do not assume the child knows. Remind the child who you are and what time or day it is.
2. *Reassuring.* Lets the child know he is safe. Even if nothing outwardly scary is taking place, the triggered child might not know he is safe. Tell the child no one is being hurt, that he is safe in the moment, not being hurt, and is okay. It can help to remind the child to breathe, or to open his eyes and look around, to feel his body and look at what he is wearing, to feel the floor under his feet. Remind the child that he is with you and is safe.
3. *Checking in.* Once the child seems more present, it can help to ask if he is okay. Does he know where he is and who you are? Some children are reassured by holding an object associated with comfort (e.g. bracelet, squeeze-ball, small toy). A drink of water or a damp cloth to wipe his face can help sometimes as well.
4. *Narrating/describing/putting in context.* Rather than asking the child what happened, you tell him (e.g. "an ambulance just went by outside with a loud siren and maybe it scared you, but we are all okay here, and no one is hurt"). The child may not remember or may have a hard time putting his feelings into words. If something happened in the school or classroom, describe it simply and without blame.
5. *Deferring blame/investigation/consequence until the child is calm.* It is important to refrain from using interrogative questions such as "Why did you do that?" and "What got into you?" The child may not know and may not

remember. Once the child is calm, reiterate what happened (he may have been unable to process it earlier). If misbehavior took place, calmly explain the cause-and-effect (e.g., "You pushed Cynthia, and when someone pushes in our class they get time-out, so please go sit in the time-out chair now") without getting into an argument. Refrain from making general statements about the child's character (e.g. "Stop lying. You always do that"). Calmly explain that even if one does not remember doing something or did not mean to do it, there is still a consequence to deal with. Be kind but firm.

6. *Providing safety for all.* The safety of everyone is paramount, adults included. If the child tends to be violent or out of control, arrange a backup plan that the child knows about ahead of time. It may mean having other adults on call (to care for other children, to help manage the child, to speak with paramedics) or other preplanned help. It helps to be prepared. That being said, in years of using the tool-kit with traumatized and overwhelmed children and adolescents, I not once had a situation escalate to unsafe when the child was offered grounding, reassured of safety, and helped in a clear, de-escalating way.

Minimizing and Handling Triggers

Minimizing Triggers

Triggers (i.e. trauma reminders) are best addressed in therapy, where they can become less activating through trauma processing. In the interim, it can help to keep everyday situations (e.g. school, field-trips, language work) as free of overwhelm as possible, because triggers disrupt a child's day and reduce availability for learning, listening, and processing. This does not mean that children can never be exposed to anything that potentially upsets them. Not only is this unrealistic but it can reinforce avoidance. Also, we may not know what triggers children until after they have already reacted, and even then we may not understand what led children to dissociate if they have amnesia to it or cannot verbalize what happened.

What we can try to do is to minimize sudden exposure to things we know are trauma reminders and prepare for those that are probable. For example, if we know that red fingernail polish triggers a child because it is a reminder of what a perpetrator had, it can help to have ours a different color, or the child could be occupied with that instead of listening or learning. If a child was mauled by a dog, a book about dogs may not be the best story choice for testing comprehension. More often, however, children do not know what scares them, are unable to explain, or are too scared to. This leave us to infer what could have triggered the child by trying to reconstruct what took place right before: Was there an unusual sound, a smell, or a change in scenery, activity, or personnel? Something someone said? Once identified, triggers can be prevented or at least handled.

Handling Triggers

Even known triggers cannot always be avoided. Handling triggers means helping children safely manage trauma reminders that are likely to occur. If a fire alarm is triggering, children may benefit from knowing about a fire drill a few minutes before it actually begins. They can be reminded what to expect and what it does and does not mean (i.e. a drill, not an actual fire), what will happen (e.g. everyone walk out quietly), and what can help them remember it is just a drill (e.g. look around, touch their bracelet, feel their friend's hand). Providing choice can help (e.g. who to walk out with), along with support through the drill to keep the child grounded. Follow-up of narrating what took place after it is over can verbalize and desensitize the experience.

Handling triggers also means helping children know that feeling scared does not need to mean awful things will happen, and they can be okay even if something 'reminded them of something scary.' Calm times are good for practicing how to recognize and what to do if they begin to 'feel not okay': ask for help, touch an item that grounds them, take a breath, take note of what they are wearing and where they are, etc. Knowing what to do can reduce helplessness and increase regulation. Speaking about handling triggers tells the child that others understand and will support them through difficult emotions (Ford & Courtois 2013, Gomez 2012, Silberg 2013, Wieland 2011, Yehuda 2011).

Noting Shifts and Pre-Shifts

One of the most helpful things adults can do for children is to note and respond to early signs of overwhelm (Cozolino 2006, 2014, Schore 2012, van der Kolk 2014)—even more so in traumatized children, who endured the intolerable and whose panic or reexperiencing can easily escalate small discomforts into overwhelm. By noticing and responding to shifts that indicate imminent overwhelm, we can help children before things become too much. Not only does this reduce loneliness, but the experience of arousal that does not overwhelm can assist with self-regulation (Gomez 2012, Loewenstein 2006, Silberg 2013, van der Kolk 2014). Narrating can help bring the child's experience into awareness and provide opportunities for practicing more options for reaction.

Every child has his or her own 'cues' for distress: acting out, shutting down, fidgeting, losing focus or becoming hyperfocused, getting suddenly sleepy, behaving immaturely, or getting clingy, whiny, or snippy. It helps to be familiar with particular children and their idiosyncrasies, but a good rule of thumb is to attend to shifts—behaviorally, emotionally, cognitively, physically, etc. Teachers and caregivers are often quite adept at noticing 'problem kids' about to "go ballistic" and note a "there he/she goes" when a student is about to act out or shut down. By understanding such cues as intervention points, adults can help a child get grounded and can assist the child in identifying precursors to overwhelm that can allow the child to seek help.

Manny sought asylum in my office. The third grader's teacher kicked him out for "classroom disturbance" (i.e. going to get water without permission), and he seethed with injustice at how other children slipped out unpunished, but him the teacher yelled at and threw out. "I almost kick the door," he sputtered, "but then I remember you say if I need to calm down I can come here to sit quiet and get calm. So I come . . ."

I praised him for remembering and for not kicking the door. Had I been in session, he would have had to sit there without disturbing, but I happened to be between sessions and let him vent what he wanted to do: scream at the teacher, break the table, "mess up the class." I was glad he did none of those and told him so, praising him for coming to tell me how he felt instead. It was no empty praise: Manny had done all that and more when mad. The fact that he remembered the option to go someplace to get calm was a big step. The boy took a deep breath, grinned bashfully, and gave me a side-hug. He then sat down to doodle quietly (and got sufficiently bored to be happy to return to the classroom by the bell).

Safety and trust are built every time we help a child not get further into a trauma state. This helps differentiate the present from the past, when there was no help and overwhelm took over. Children who feel better understood and heard can calm more quickly at the adult's voice and/or presence. This mirrors what takes place normally when an infant calms at the sound of a caregiver's approach: The association of care reinforces regulation and security (Cozolino 2006, van der Kolk 2014). It is a mutually beneficial dyad: As the child responds by calming, the adult feels more capable and more available to help.

Reinforcing Safety

Safety is essential for connection, learning, and exploration. We establish safety with newborns when we hold them securely, and through our sensitive response to their needs (Cozolino 2006, Gaensbauer 2011, van der Kolk 2014). Feeling safe allows babies to be curious. It gives them a secure base from which to move and relate without fear of hurt and pain. If safety is shaken, exploration ceases. Curiosity stops. Wary babies bury their faces in caregivers' necks and burrow into holding arms. If their fear stays unrelieved, they cry, shake, or shut down (Bowlby 1997, Lyons-Ruth & Block 1996, Scaer 2014, van der Kolk 2014).

Trauma makes safety a tricky thing even if external safety is established or assumed restored (e.g. an adoptive home, the health crisis being over). Even if we believe that children are safe, they may not feel safe (Silberg 2013, Wieland 2011). If their security was disrupted repeatedly (e.g. multiple foster-homes), they might keep anticipating another rupture. This can remain even after (sometimes especially after) a long stay in a stable home, where a child may believe rupture to be increasingly imminent (Bruning 2007, Smith et al 1998). Other children never had security and have no sense of what 'safe' is (Albers et al 2005, Miller 2005). Children may wait for inevitable abuse (or try to provoke it to alleviate anticipatory anxiety). They may not know how to recognize, trust, or relax in the knowledge that they are cared for.

Verbalizing and reassurance of safety is important. This may include repeated stating of safe boundaries as well as use of things like the tool-kit whenever trauma reminders come up. Safety can be bolstered by planning ahead and providing some measure of control. For example, if a medically traumatized child requires a procedure, it may help to explain what to expect, let the child ask questions, and involve the child in decisions (e.g. what small toy to bring, who the child prefers to be with at the time of the procedure) (Kuttner 2010). Familiar objects can reduce disorientation. Prearranged hand cues or flip-cards can minimize panic in a child who may not be able to speak (e.g. breathing tube). A sense of safety can be increased by informing medical personnel of the child's needs and ways of grounding.

For some children, attaining safety is hard because their reality reflects lack of it. They might still be shuttled through the foster-system. Children can be pulled between divorced parents and not know to whom they need to show allegiance. There can be instability at home or ongoing medical procedures. They can be (rightfully) wary and dismissive, unable to feel truly safe. However, establishing 'islands of safety' is still important, and being even 'slightly less' unsafe can help. Ensuring safety—in whatever scope and contexts possible—can teach children that safety is possible, that some people care, that they matter, and that there is hope.

Keeping Teens Informed

Much of what applies to children still applies to adolescents, but traumatized teens deserve special attention. Many have accumulated more trauma and have had to manage overwhelm (and apply coping skills) longer. Their language and communication issues may seem less pronounced compared with younger children's, in part because teens often hide difficulties under indifference, withdrawal, aggression, or confrontation. Their behaviors often mask and deflect away from shame, guilt, anxiety, frustration, helplessness, and low self-esteem, and they can come across as inflexible and distrusting. If nothing else, this makes it even more important that we help them know we understand.

Traumatized teens need as much reassurance, safety, comfort, and connection as younger children do, but they are not simply bigger versions and require developmentally appropriate assistance. Explanations and reassurance may still need to be simplified, but should never be infantilized: Many traumatized teens already feel defective and are hypersensitive to being talked down to or 'dumbed down.' Adolescents straddle the fence between childhood and adulthood, need and independence, immaturity and maturity, and teen years are sensitive and turbulent under the best of conditions. They are often even more so for children who enter adolescence with traumatized regulatory systems and compromised communication.

Traumatized teens often feel unreal and/or perceive the world around them as fake, but may not know how to verbalize these perceptions and might not attempt to if they believe it makes them weird or different (Lehman 2005). Psychoeducation and normalization (e.g. about trauma reactions, how some level of derealization and depersonalization is common in teenagers) can be reassuring and help them feel less isolated and not as crazy (Silberg 2013, Steinberg & Schnall 2000, van der Hart et al 2006, Wieland 2011). Adolescents I worked with were relieved that things they had believed were so different and wrong about themselves were actually normal responses to abnormal situations. They found it helpful to reframe distressing realities such as feeling numb, being unaware of things they did, and struggling to word experiences as coping skills that were outdated rather than wrong. It felt empowering to them to see posttraumatic responses not only as explainable, but as lifesaving, and to realize that they had found ways to manage in impossible situations. They judged themselves less and trusted their ability to manage even better now that they had help.

Boundaries, Honesty, and Being 'Real'

Autonomy is important for all adolescents and even more so for those whose autonomy was compromised and who are justifiably oversensitive to fake choices, implied blame, and double-binds. Teenagers need to feel that they have real choices and are not 'done to.' Trust is a fragile thing for people who experienced betrayal (Herman 1997, Howell 2011, Freyd & Birrell 2013, van der Hart et al 2006, Wallin 2007). It is especially so for traumatized teens, whose skepticism was honed by betrayal and is fueled by the developmental tasks of doubting and reassessing truth and reality (Silberg 2013). They will hold adults to a (sometimes unreasonably) high standard and deserve that we at least be truthful. Adolescents whose truth and boundaries were compromised have every reason to doubt people's motives, and maintaining scrupulously clear and respectful boundaries (and consequences) is paramount.

I have learned: Do not say one thing and do another. Keep communication open to repair any breakdown or accidental boundary breach. Be ready to be tested. Be honest but nonburdening about your feelings. Admit errors. Difficult conversations are opportunities. Be real. Listen. Explain. Interpersonal communication is the hallmark of teen years, which makes every interaction a chance to rebuild what trauma broke.

15 Communication Intervention for Traumatized Children

The increased risk for overwhelm in children who have delays and disabilities (Benedict et al 1990, Crosse et al 1993, Goldson 1998, Sullivan & Knutson 2000), combined with the impact of trauma on development (see Part 3) means that essentially all child professionals have seen or currently see traumatized children. It is obviously important for communication-disorders clinicians (speech-language pathologists and audiologists) to be aware of the ways communication and trauma interact, but it is relevant for anyone working with children. Trauma awareness does not mean one does psychotherapy or "trauma work" (see Chapter 17 for scope of practice issues). Rather, it calls for identifying and minimizing trauma reactions and for improving communication so a child can make use of interventions.

While the approaches described in this chapter all fall within the scope of practice of speech-language pathologists, many will be familiar to other child professionals, too. They involve utilizing existing clinical skills in a trauma-aware way that takes into account the 'holes' that trauma rents in children's affective, relational, and communicative world. Depending on the children, their age, their circumstances, and how they coped, therapeutic strategies may involve establishing safety and grounding, reciprocal dyads, and play. Strategies often include building and expanding vocabulary (e.g. for state language), addressing causation and sequence, modeling narrative and discourse skills, and managing symbolic language and social interaction. Intervention may address language *content* (nouns, verbs, descriptive words, pronouns, prepositions, temporal terms, etc.), *form* (sentence structure, word inflections, tenses, etc.), and *use* (pragmatics, turn-taking, communicative intents, context and listeners' knowledge, social cues, symbolic language/expressions, humor, etc.)

Safety and availability for learning are prerequisites for any therapeutic interaction. This chapter may be especially relevant to speech-language pathologists but is meant to offer direction to anyone who deals with traumatized children. The clinical suggestions are not meant as a comprehensive or hierarchical list—various aspects often combine in every session—and are detailed separately only for the sake of clinical clarity.

Offering Compassion and Grounding

Compassion and kindness regulate stress and are communicated in words, facial expressions, and safe affection (Cozolino 2006, 2014, Siegel 2012, van der Kolk 2014). Children learn that they matter when we note their distress and calm it; when we understand them and offer doable solutions; when we model empathy and refrain from blame and shame; when we communicate our happiness about them and praise what is admirable. Children who experienced trauma can have difficulty letting in kindness, especially if it has been missing, sparse, or misinterpreted. They may not recognize kindness or be too activated or shut down to make use of it. They may believe kindness comes with strings attached or that they do not deserve it. Yet it is imperative that we be kind.

This means addressing behaviors and their consequences with firm fairness and empathy that takes into account how children act out from places of anger, helplessness, and pain and need guidance, not judgment. Persistent misbehavior may be communicating unmet needs: hunger for attention, connection, acceptance, affection, or needing a break. It may signal overwhelm or be 'testing' whether care is indeed available. Traumatized children had no choice but to manage overwhelm and helplessness. They need help to learn to be grounded and that it can be safe for their feelings to be seen and heard while they learn new ways to communicate and regulate.

Grounding

Traumatized children may not know what it means to be calmly grounded, especially if they dissociate preemptively or oscillate between hypervigilance and shutting down. Practicing grounding and calming can help children be 'in their bodies' more. It increases their availability for learning as well as the effectiveness of cues like the 'tool-kit' (see previous chapter) when they get activated. Calming stress activation is necessary for the language centers and executive functions to work, and children often benefit from practice at grounding at the beginning of sessions. I may use variations of "noticing exercises" (a deliberately mild term not commonly associated with fear), which often incorporate some language work:

- 'Noticing' when a sound starts or stops (e.g. musical chairs), taking turns producing sounds (noise-makers, music player, vocally) for the other to notice starting/stopping.
- Throwing and catching a ball, including variations of throwing lightly, slowly, fast, high-low, etc.
- Looking in the mirror and having children touch their arm/knee/head/etc. to notice how it feels. The visual and tactile information helps make this an integrated process.

- Taking turns in "Simon says" (more about this task later in the chapter). Movement helps regulation and it takes awareness and attention to follow or provide directions.
- "All Senses" game: noticing air going in/out during breathing, feet on the floor, sounds in and outside the room, things one sees, smells, tastes; identifying items by their texture; noticing warm/cool/smooth/rough/soft/hard.
- Taking turns blowing air out and noticing how a cotton ball moves on one's palm; playing 'cotton-ball-derby' to blow the cotton ball off the table (helps parasympathetic calming, concentration, body and breath control).
- Blowing onto a small mirror and noticing the fog on it (note: some children may not want to look at their own faces), fogging the whole mirror or just a streak, etc.
- Noticing and slowing down breathing—tapping or 'counting fingers' as the breath goes in, humming on the out—can reduce autonomic nervous system activation and can help children's bodies 'remember' what to do when they get upset.
- Noticing scents. If you find ones the child enjoys, spray it on a tissue/handkerchief to help the child get grounded when activated.
- Squeezing a stress-ball and noticing how the palm feels, the movement of the fingers, and the 'give' of the toy. Noticing differences between items in alternating palms.
- Listening to different types of music and noticing where in their bodies they feel it, what it makes them want to do (jump, dance, sleep, smile). Put music that helps the child's body 'quiet down calmly' onto a portable player for times the child gets upset (note: don't assume 'familiar' nursery rhymes are okay—some can be triggering).

Modeling Attachment-Reinforcing Communication Dyads

Reciprocity

The myriad ways we note actions and reactions in those around us and they in us form the foundation for social connection, regulation, and learning. Traumatized children may miss opportunities for learning how to do so and frequently need help with reciprocity. With very young children, this may mean revisiting peek-a-boo and finger-play, alternating turns with noise-makers, swinging (and wanting to be pushed again), playing ball, building and dismantling towers from blocks, hiding and finding objects (note: some children may get triggered by hide-and-seek). Reciprocity work in older children can involve playing catch or Cat's Cradle; taking turns in "Simon says"; and playing board games, question-and-answer games, and riddles and definitions (e.g. I Spy); alternating song lines; and reading scripts.

Singing and Rhythm

We are 'wired' for rhythm: Fetuses hear their mother's heartbeat and body rhythms, and our nervous system remains attuned to rhythm through the interplay of our own heartbeat and autonomic system (Nazzi et al 1998, Ninio & Snow 1996, Schore 2012, van der Kolk 2014). Lullaby singing, back patting, and baby-rocking are universal ways for calming little ones, and rhythm remains comforting to not so little ones as well. Dance, choir, chanting, clapping, rocking, and swaying are integral to rituals of healing, community, and connection worldwide and throughout the lifespan (Konner 2010, van der Kolk 2014). Newborns are soothed and reassured by the humming, pacing, and bouncing by caregivers. Rhythm continues in nursery rhymes and finger-play, rope-skipping, hopscotch, etc. It assists with planning and coordinating, helps academic instruction through tapping syllables, rhyming, pauses in sentences, and more. Rhythm supports speech fluency and remains a way of connection and comfort well after cognitive skills may be diminished by illness and dementia.

Trauma can leave children disconnected from the soothing of others (though the need is so basic that children may rock themselves). Even in children who had a baseline of soothing, overwhelm can disrupt integration of body and sound, connection and calm. Practicing breath, tempo, movement, and sound during calm interactions can establish and reinforce pathways to support regulation during less calm times.

Manuel (see Chapter 10*) was adopted from an orphanage, and his adoptive mother worried he was autistic. Though thirteen months old, aspects of him felt "like newborn." He vocalized little. He also rocked for hours in self-soothing. His parents understood he needed comfort but could not bear him rocking alone. Rocking with him still got him "glassy-eyed." I recommended rocking side-to-side while singing to him, and modeled it by holding Manuel in my lap on my physioball. He soon relaxed into me and when I stopped, he looked up in a precursor of anticipation. His parents purchased a similar ball, then installed a hammock for more side-to-side rocking. Manuel loved it. The movement was familiarly soothing but different enough from the dissociating motion to allow engagement rather than isolation. He began to climb onto his parents' lap and initiate a side-to-side rocking motion in 'request.' He vocalized more—first during mutual rocking and then in other interactions. The hammock became a bonding routine. It provided the boy with holding, physical contact, and the calming vibrations of his parents' heartbeat and voice as they sang to him. In therapy we introduced peek-a-boo and pat-a-cake and many other interactive finger-play games, along with daily routines, books, and songs. Manuel became better regulated and increasingly available for learning and play. He began pointing for things and babbling, soon followed by words. By age 2:6 Manuel was a curious toddler rapidly closing communication and language gaps.*

Rocking in a hammock may not work with all children—it may be inappropriate for some children or offer too much proximity. However, other shared activities can help caregivers repair some of the lack of attunement that trauma and maltreatment represent:

- Rocking or swinging with the child while humming or singing softly. Modeling with a stuffed toy can be helpful in some children (choose a different direction than that of self-soothing, which can trigger dissociation)
- Making time for cuddling—even with older children. They may not sit in one's lap, but they can still sit together, share a swing, hold hands, give hugs, put a head on a shoulder—whatever proximity the child is comfortable with. Safe affection is especially important in children who were abused and may not have a baseline for safe touch (more on touch in Chapter 14)
- Playing pat-a-cake and other rhythmic games (jump rope, hopscotch, catch with a ball)
- Singing and playing music together
- Moving and dancing to music—letting the child 'choreograph'
- Chanting, humming, skating, walking, and other repetitive activities
- Doing yoga or martial arts together

Play Schemes and Symbolization

Going Back to Basics

Children need help 'filling in' the holes that trauma and posttraumatic activation created. Going back to basics to strengthen their foundation is important so they will not be 'tripped' by weak points. This can mean different things in different children. For a child who had limited experience with asking questions, it can include basic question/answer skills, exploring opinions, offering suggestions, finding preferences, identifying motives, and so on. In children who lacked opportunities to initiate, there can be reciprocal activities, communication expectation, and problem solving. A child who struggles with listening may need discrimination and identification activities, following directions, auditory memory games, sustained attention tasks, and so on. A child who struggles with symbolic representation or discourse may benefit from modeled play schemes and narratives. Most traumatized children can use help with noting and identifying body language and emotions, humor and the absurd, refusal and assent.

Revisiting vulnerable aspects of communication is essential because it helps children experience less error, confusion, or misunderstanding and establishes skills for varied tasks and interactions. Some tasks may seem trivial, but to overlook basic skills because a child seems "too old for this kind of stuff" can miss the very fundamentals the child needs.

"Everyone Tired"—Marcy: The Dissociating Power of Overwhelm

Marcy was Miss Passive. Rarely disruptive, the eight-year-old just did not listen. "She's a butt in the seat with no one home," the teacher said. Marcy spoke little, initiated less, and showed very limited interest in academic or social activities. She was neither happy nor reluctant. Life skirted her by. She rarely described or added her opinion, and her narrative was bare and practically devoid of affect words. Questions about cause and effect, motive, or sequential order stumped her and she struggled following directions, let alone predicting a next step. "I feel like shaking her up," the teacher admitted. "This kid needs to wake up!" I wondered about Marcy's lassitude. I knew little about her home life. She looked cared-for and lived with her mother and twin toddler siblings in the housing project where many children in the school lived. She had few friends and fewer interests, seeming apathetic and away, unavailable for engaging.

There is no learning without engagement. To "shake her up" Na'ama style, we tossed a ball across the auditorium stage, clapped rhythms, and played variations of "Simon says" at the beginning of every session. I found out Marcy liked Britney Spears and brought some of her songs. We sang "Oops I Did It Again," danced some of the moves, and organized a 'concert' with toy figurines. We elaborated what they 'might have done' before/during/after the concert: gotten dressed, chosen what to eat, stood in line for the bathroom. I modeled body states (e.g. hungry, tired, thirsty, sick) and emotions (e.g. excited, worried, happy, disappointed, scared) in the toys and the stories we made up for them. Marcy was not exactly enthusiastic but she seemed more alert than in class and occasionally initiated or 'corrected' me. The first time I saw her laugh was when I forgot some moves and substituted them for silliness.

We expanded the concert theme to other 'outings' for the figurines. I took photos of some of the settings Marcy arranged and we added short 'stories' to accompany them: the doll being sick, a birthday party, baking cookies, visiting the zoo. To tie things to the real world, I brought cookies and milk, a wrapped present, things to experience. Marcy began to offer her opinion, she dictated what the figurines were doing and how they felt.

As her ability to identify and describe body states improved and her narrative expanded, Marcy also began sharing more about her own experience. She was less shut down but seemed sadder. "Today everyone tired," she stated one day after our brief ball game. She laid the toys in a pile in the box, looking exhausted herself. "You seem tired, too," I noted gently and she looked at me in some alarm. I could almost see her awareness flicker. "It is okay, Marcy," I reassured. "You can be however you need to be here. Nothing bad is happening. You are here in the Speech room with me." She blinked and reached for my hand, and I squeezed hers softly. Marcy had begun to take my hand during our 'dance routines' and I was glad she felt comfortable to initiate. She took a deep breath. "I am tired," she whispered, "from people in my house."

She said nothing more about it that day but shared more in following sessions. First just that she was tired. Then about someone called "John" at home at night; then that there were actually several such 'Johns,' all strangers who 'cussed' at her mom and 'were scary' and 'nasty' and made Marcy 'feel not okay' and 'want to go away.' I alerted Child Protective Services about suspected risk. They found that Marcy's mother was 'entertaining men' to support a narcotic addiction. There was strong indication Marcy and possibly her siblings were molested.

This had been going on for quite some time but Marcy was too shut down to speak earlier and did not know how to verbalize or name fatigue, wariness, disgust, or fear. Her lethargy was partially physical (she was getting very little sleep) and partially protective (she could not escape her circumstances other than by shutting down). Filling in the basics meant providing opportunities for her to be in her body and giving meaning to verbalizing and narrating. Maybe it helped her find the energy and words to tell what she was enduring and needed help with.

Incorporating Body States and Emotive States

Trauma belies words, and language centers get shut down by overwhelm, making it difficult to process events (van der Kolk 2014). Children often cope with overwhelm by dissociating, numbing their bodies and pushing away affect and its meaning. When their emotions and body states during trauma remain non-verbalized, their experience—intentionally or not—can end up misunderstood, minimized, distorted, or ignored. All this makes it difficult for children to connect events, emotions, and body states.

Being grounded allows us to be aware of sensations and feelings that inform us of our needs: go to the bathroom, get a drink, ask for a break, request help, seek comfort, etc. Children are still acquiring the ability to note and respond to these cues and are especially vulnerable to the impact of dissociation. Traumatized children may need help not only with comprehending the meaning of the words for body states and emotions, but with the very experience of identifying and managing sensations, reactions, and feelings. They require opportunities to connect emotive language and body states with contexts, situations, feelings, sensations, and words.

Traumatized children may sometimes use words to describe feelings and states. This may not mean that they truly understand those concepts or are describing their experiences. Some children look for cues from others as to what they should say. They may not know how to communicate their own perceptions, lack the words, or be too scared. Marcy could not say she was exhausted and afraid until she made the connection between what fatigue was and the sensations in her own body. She knew 'tired, angry, hungry, excited' had meanings and could apply them in some contexts, but the concepts were not connected to her own experience and so she did not use them in relation to herself.

Being able to identify and name affect and body states requires situational awareness, comprehension of context, and self-awareness for recognizing one's sensations and emotions. Traumatized children may find it easier to 'read' facial expressions and body language in others than to name their own, especially for feelings that are difficult. Children may not want to admit being angry if they believe it makes them 'bad.' They may not admit affection if feeling it (or the need for it) may imply danger or risk rejection. We need to model and provide varied opportunities with neutral as well as more emotionally laden contexts for children to practice identifying, labeling, and describing emotions and body states in others and in themselves.

Teaching affective language can include:

- Teaching body states through play, modeling, interaction, and stories
- Using "intensity charts" to help quantify the 'volume' or 'how much of the feeling' they may have (e.g. pale yellow through to bright orange; a chart of numbers from 0 to 10, with 10 being the 'loudest/strongest')
- Exploring situations, characters, and motivations
- Providing specific affective vocabulary in words and illustrations (e.g. hopeful, disappointed, cranky, frustrated, rude, confused), as well as state and affective range (e.g. uncomfortable, achy, in pain; irritated, annoyed, angry, enraged; pleased, happy, ecstatic)
- Using current events, media photos, body language, and depicted emotions in cartoons, books, movies, and everyday situations, along with gentle exploration of the child's feelings, opinions, and views

Generalization—Too Much, Too Little

Learning a new concept often involves initial overgeneralization and/or undergeneralization. Infants often attribute a word to too few or too many items before they 'map' its semantic meaning (Dromi 1987). They may call all men "daddy" but use "bottle" only for their milk bottle, call all colors "red," or use colors interchangeably before they realize that each hue has a name. Concepts are learned through practice and the feedback from others, which helps children ascertain whether they have gotten it right or not.

Traumatized children often have less opportunity for practicing new concepts. They can be too occupied to attend, wary about testing hypotheses, and have less tolerance for trial-and-error. They may misinterpret others' reactions or overgeneralize or undergeneralize: any frown or lack of praise as being angry with them, all refusals as 'scary' or 'mean' (Heller & Lapierre 2012, Nadeau et al 2013, Shields & Cicchetti 1998, Silberg 2013, Wieland 2011). Traumatized children may use a lot of "I don't know," "I forgot," "Nothing," and "I don't care" or may always be "fine," "mad," or "okay." Repetition and experience in varied contexts may be needed before they can incorporate a concept into their world. Other traumatized children use very specific or highly dramatic words for describing relatively neutral events and need opportunity to learn 'gradients' of concepts.

Usage errors carry information about things children are unclear about, as well as things they are trying to tell us but we may be missing. An "I'm starving" from a child who just had a snack may just be an exaggeration. He may also believe that anything short of starving is unworthy of request, or that for him, even a trace of hunger triggers much worse (see Mika's story later in this chapter).

Conceptualizing How-to

When a child seems to have an unusual perception of a word, it can help to teach it in a tiered way. For example, the concept of 'happy':

- Using everyday contexts for describing how you (or a toy) experience it: what makes you happy; how it feels in your body; what it makes you want to do (e.g. smile)
- Presenting it in varied contexts and strengths (e.g. people feel happy getting something they wanted, being understood, feeling liked, going to Disney World, etc.; one can be a 'little happy' or 'the happiest ever')
- Exploring the opposite/s of the concept: what "sad" may mean to you or in a story and how 'opposite' is not necessarily absence (i.e. sad is not 'not happy' but has its own quality and contexts)
- Teaching how feelings can coexist: You can be happy that there is no school and bored from missing friends; happy that Mom is around all day but sad that she is sick
- Practicing the concept in neutral and controlled contexts, before using it in relation to the child's history (note of caution: see scope of practice limits in next chapter)
- Checking repeatedly for preconceptions—the concept may not mean the same to the child in new or loaded contexts

Sequence and Consequence

"He Is the Best Little Patient in the World"—Liam: The Price of Assumption

Liam was five when he came to see me for articulation issues. Born healthy, he developed bowel issues and needed a colonoscopy and rectal biopsy at age four. His parents thought he handled the preparation and testing very well. "Probably doesn't remember any of it," they told me during intake. Liam had diet restrictions and was diligent about keeping them. His parents interpreted his adherence as being mature about his issues but admitted he was "somewhat overfocused" on his diet. Overfocused was an understatement: Liam was suspicious of anything I prepared for oral-motor exercises, and even though I assured him that I had carefully followed his dietary restrictions, he still demanded to see and have ingredient lists read to him by me or his embarrassed parents.

Language was not the primary reason Liam came to see me, but his rigidity reflected difficulties with causation, sequence, pragmatics, and ambiguity. I explained what we were doing and why (e.g. tongue movements that prepared for tongue-tip sounds). He enjoyed explanations, yet struggled to comprehend how an exercise could be for more than one thing or could be done in varied order, arguing 'it had to be' one way. I added cause/effect games and sequence stories and we 'thought up' multiple possibilities of "what happens next." We 'experimented' with how the same ingredient could be in different things (e.g. milk in ice cream, cheese, and yogurt), and 'found out' how various things can be drawn from the same shape (e.g. circle: sun, face, flower, orange, clock). His parents continued at home: What can be done with an orange? Does it matter what cup you pour juice into? What things are made of wood? Which are soft/hard/square? Liam soon caught on and his rigidity relaxed, though not with food.

A few weeks into therapy, when he still asked to see the ingredient list, I noted, "It must be tiring to worry so much about people maybe giving you something you're not supposed to eat."

Liam sighed, "I have to."

I asked how come, and he stated: "Because it's my fault if I get sick and break my tummy."

His father stared at him, shocked. "None of it is your fault, champ. Your tummy is great now. Also Mommy and I always tell people ahead of time . . ."

Liam shook his head. "What if they forget, Daddy? I don't want the doctor to find more junk food in my tummy and get mad and hurt my bum."

A year prior, when Liam's parents told him he needed to "drink the medicine" for the doctors to look at his tummy and make him better, Liam got confused. The medicine didn't make him feel better. It made him feel yucky and his tummy hurt more. When they went to the hospital (for the colonoscopy), Liam thought that maybe he "broke the medicine" by eating Cheez Doodles his daddy sometimes let him have "as a little secret between us boys" but which his mommy always said were "junk food" and "bad for his tummy." Liam was scared to ask if the Cheez Doodles broke the medicine because he didn't want the doctor to be angry and he didn't want more medicine. Then he was in a bed and felt "not good," but his parents smiled like everything was fine and told him that the doctors "checked his tummy." Liam was confused—he didn't see the doctor check his tummy. Also his head felt sleepy and his 'bum' hurt and though his parents didn't explain, he heard them talk with Papa and Nana and say it was for "finding out." They went home without the doctor making his tummy better and Liam thought he did something wrong. His bum felt tender. Maybe the doctor found out the secret junk food Cheez Doodles in his tummy where his bum was and it was his fault that he was feeling yucky and his tummy hurt.

Liam was given dietary restrictions. The diet helped but he needed follow-up and returned to the hospital for a CT and other tests. The four-year-old boy never put up a fuss. He let the doctors place IVs, palpate his abdomen, test for allergies, and check him rectally. His mother was proud and said he was "the best little patient in the world." She did not realize that Liam was "being good" because he was terrified. He believed he needed to make sure he didn't "break his tummy again." Sensing that his "tummy issues" were somewhat embarrassing to his parents, he also felt ashamed and guilty. He tried very hard to "only be good" and to be clean and "not get tummy germs." He became hyperanxious about his dietary restrictions and pho-bic of 'junk food.' He avoided friends' houses because maybe food would not be okay, maintained a perimeter around him during lunch, and cried if a child touched him without washing hands after a snack, claiming that "it will hurt my tummy and it will make me sick."

Liam could not verbalize his perceptions and how he felt until he was able to manage cause-and-effect in other, neutral contexts. That experience allowed him to let in reassurance that his belief about what happened was not the only expla-nation and to ask questions about what he had assumed to be reality. He became less worried about food or germs and his parents asked the doctor to explain what the test did and how some of the food restrictions were only temporary. We wrote up his 'tummy story' and Liam put a drawing of himself at the end of it, looking happy and healthy and strong (more on stories later in this chapter).

Breaking It Down

Young children often find causation in disconnected things and may fail to see connections where they do exist. They are even more prone to errors when they are overwhelmed or dissociated, or if events truly do not add up or are left unex-plained. Traumatized children may need assistance with identifying and under-standing causation, responsibility, culpability, and consequence:

- Breaking events into their components; organizing schedules into different activities; dissecting long directions into single steps; parsing assignments into doable steps.
- Ensuring children comprehend what happened and what will take place, what their responsibilities are, what behaviors/actions are expected or what to expect.
- Depicting sequences in multisensory ways to help internalize the concept of connection (puzzle pieces, paper-chains, etc.). Visual schedules, pictured steps, flow-charts, preview, and review can scaffold understanding. For older chil-dren, notes and bullets, lists and highlights, storylines and keywords can help.
- As they improve, a 'step' can represent several mini-steps that no longer need to be separated.

- Visible cues (e.g. numbers, arrows) can help children get oriented: what they did already, what took place, what is next, and after that; what is gone; what to expect.
- Visual scaffolding can also help reorient and reinforce grounding for children who are dissociated, so they can see where they left off, resume an activity, and know what to complete.

Predicting the Very Predictable

Understanding our world and what things mean helps us trust that we would know when we can relax or must act. Trauma often leaves children in perpetual anticipation of overwhelm, which disrupts processing and keeps children hypervigilant or preemptively shut down (van der Kolk 2014). Because helplessness is intolerable, children may grab onto whatever they think has predictive value and become anxious with any associations. Others go numb and miss real clues to what is about to take place, only to feel startled and confused. Feeling helpless in a capricious world adds stress, and traumatized children can oscillate from bossy to apathetic, raging to numb, needy to stoic (Silberg 2013, Waters 2005, Wieland 2011).

In order to help children be present, grounded, and able to learn, we need to minimize helplessness—for example, prompting before anticipated changes, explaining what might take place, and reviewing it later to address misconceptions and assure comprehension. Most third graders do not need to be told that the jarring bell will be that of a fire drill, or about an upcoming change of classroom. However, for some children, this can make the difference between staying grounded or dissociating. I found it best to err on the side of redundancy and let the children tell me when they don't need it anymore.

Checking in—Not Assuming Comprehension

Children who are hypervigilant or shut down miss instruction. They may only 'get' snippets of what is said. Also, even if they seem relatively calm now, they may be unable to connect things said now with what they were told earlier if they had not been as calm at the time. Trauma disrupts integrative skills (Scaer 2014, Schore 2012, van der Kolk 2014).

- Limiting errors of misunderstanding—checking in to see that children understood directions before they attempt a task. Children can repeat or show what they understood about what they need to do.
- Double-checking symbolic language, metaphors, ambiguous words, pun, and jokes.
- Teaching expressions ahead of time or stopping to review and explain them.

- Not assuming that children know an expression even if they have heard it before: They might not remember, it might have been a different context or setting, or they might have been too overwhelmed to 'get it.'
- Explaining and practicing humor and jokes. I often teach some as we explore what's funny and what makes it so.
- Finding the difference between funny and cruel, silly and crude, appropriate and rude.

The Meaning of 'Why,' 'How,' and 'When'

Traumatic experiences can be incomprehensible, unpredictable, illogical, and overwhelming (Herman 1997). Time concepts get distorted in trauma (Terr 1983), and are tricky for children as it is—let alone for a child who dissociates and 'loses time' or whose life lacks predictability and reference to schedule or time. Traumatic memory can be scrambled (Brewin 2005), with multiple traumas mixing so that aspects of events mesh together to further confuse time. Being triggered makes children feel—psychologically and/or physiologically—like it is happening again, mixing past and present. Difficulties with 'why,' 'how,' and 'when' can extend to nontrauma situations, too. Understanding what is happening and why can help reduce confusion and improve grounding, and traumatized children benefit from modeling and scaffolding of causation, procedure, timing, and sequence concepts:

- With young children: providing tangible opportunities to manipulate items and modeled narration of why, because, how, and when (e.g. wondering what would happen if a cup is tilted, why the juice spilled, what to do next, reviewing what happened and why; revisiting it the following day to remember "what happened yesterday with the juice," etc.)
- In older children: suggesting and discussing causation in everyday events (how and why the teacher reacted to someone being silly, how to get from A to B or get a task done, what steps are necessary, why would something work or not)
- Adolescents: preplanning tasks, discussing how to manage possible delays and problems, and conceptualizing solutions (e.g. work not likely to take place during a vacation and so divide a task into fewer days; what happens if they procrastinate—anxiety, pressure, mistakes; what if they don't get the task done—loss of privilege, lesser grade)
- Calendars can anchor experiences and be visual aids for noting upcoming events, teaching time words and predictability (e.g. plans for tomorrow, field trip next week, chess club every Tuesday), reviewing past events (e.g. what happened last Monday), and looking ahead
- Photos and notes can become reminders for time, place, and cause (who came to the party last month, went to summer camp, needed their tonsils out)

Possible and Probable—Not Always What You Think

What we expect or find plausible depends on what our experiences have been and our assumptions about the world and people in it. Babies who get comforted when they cry learn it is probable that comfort will follow crying, but those who get hit for crying may learn that crying is likely to bring on more pain. A child who was abandoned without explanation may believe that someone leaving the room means losing that person forever. A child may be inconsolable if a trip is postponed, believing it will never happen. A child who had to provide 'return favors' may do something inappropriate after being praised.

Probability and plausibility in maltreating homes can be very different than those of school, therapy, or a foster-home. Traumatized children follow the 'logic' they managed to extract from incomprehensible situations but may not be able to explain why they believe what they believe. Errors and misbehaviors may not reflect a child's dysfunction but our misunderstanding of the realities and rules they are working from. We need to remain attentive to the child's reactions and demeanor, so that we can detect mismatched assumptions, and take care to explain boundaries and expectations: what they mean and why; what will or will not follow; what the child should and should not do and in what way.

Scaffolding—Working in Multimodalities

Sensory Integration and Being in the Body

Traumatic stress disrupts processing, fragments events, and changes how experiences are remembered (Brewin 2005, Gaensbauer 2002, Herman 1997, van der Kolk 2014). Because children are still learning how to integrate experiences, trauma can lead to difficulties with sensory integration, modulation, and regulation (see Chapter 6). We can help provide the child with opportunities to bridge experience across modalities, states, and senses and weave verbalization and meaning into the experiences:

- Identifying and naming how it feels to be grounded versus 'spacey,' attentive versus distracted, calm/excited/nervous/bored/tired
- Recognizing comfort and discomfort; attending to, modeling, and verbalizing the cues that bodies (and their own bodies) give. For example, when bored—do they fidget, feel sleepy?
- Incorporating activities and turn-taking for modeling and reinforcing sensory aspects of concepts like speed, intensity, loudness, balance, left-and-right, movement and stillness (e.g. walk slowly, run fast; whisper, shout; stand still, jump; hop on one foot, then the other; push, nudge, touch, tug gently, pull hard; blink, squint, peer, stare)

- Experiencing and wording sensations (ticklish, prickly, rough, smooth, soft, pointy, sharp, sticky, cold, warm)
- Grading sensations by intensity (e.g. barely heard to too loud), preference and tolerance and how these change between people and in different times (does goo feel nice or yucky? Is wool comfortable or scratchy? What flavors taste best?—go together? do not?)

Connecting the Dots—Seeing, Hearing, Touching, Feeling

Optimal learning integrates multisensory experience with narrative in context. These are the very things that stress disrupts, and traumatized children often live disjointed experiences. By helping children stay grounded for sensory experience, and giving them opportunities to process input from different senses and narrate it, children can form templates for experience and description:

- 'Scanning' and naming sensations and descriptors for seeing, smelling, hearing, tasting, touching, feeling, and thinking in everyday experiences. For example, at snack: What the apple looks like (kids' answers: "circle," "like a ball," "red with spots," "shiny," "like smiles"—i.e. sliced), feels like ("hard/wet/cold/slippery"), smells like ("wet/like apple juice . . ."), tastes like ("sweet/sour/yummy"), how it feels in your hand ("like a baseball/not heavy/easy/slippy"), to chew a bite ("crunchy/noisy/bumpy in my throat")
- Noting what is taking place around oneself: the feel of one's seat in the chair, feet on the floor (or not . . .), noises outside, visuals around the room
- Revisiting activities: drawing a picture or using a photo and/or objects to remember how it felt (e.g. a seashell and a beach photo to discuss a trip to the beach: the sounds, the sun on one's face, the sand, the seagulls, whoosh of the waves, etc.)
- Comparing and contrasting activities/events/episodes: noting similarities and differences, rating (e.g. best to worst, most to least favorite, noisiest to most quiet, most fun to most boring). Detailing differences and how they feel (e.g. kid: "the science teacher is nice and I feel calm, but the math teacher screams a lot and it feels tight in my ears")

Modifying "Simon Says"—Mindful Directions

Following directions is an everyday reality that traumatized children can find challenging. Many are diagnosed with attention issues, struggle with memory, can find directions scary, and worry about mistakes. Taking turns with directions allows children to practice how to attend to and follow directions, as well as how to initiate, formulate directions, manage mistakes, and attend to boundaries. It teaches to take turns, wait, attend to others, note and correct mistakes, rephrase and fix communication failures, initiate and respond. Alternating directions allows modeling for the difference between request, direction, suggestion, command, and appropriate and inappropriate directions. Children learn what is possible and what is not, what makes directions too hard (e.g. too long) and how to simplify, ways to ask for clarification and tolerate errors in themselves and others, even how to be silly. Role-playing can teach the difference between settings, speakers, play, and work.

I use variations on the "Simon says" theme both 1:1 and in bigger groups (e.g. family game, peers) as means for incorporating movement and grounding with attending and communication. It is a fun game, but I stay attentive to the child's reactions and responses: Trauma is experienced through the body, and some directions can be triggering or otherwise distressing. It is easy to understand that to "pretend to hit someone" or "make a scared face" might be triggering for an abused child. However, even relatively neutral directions like "close your eyes," "turn around," and "open your mouth" can remind of trauma. Directions involving touch can become confusing, especially if they include being touched or touching others.

I stay mindful not only when I am the one giving the directions but also when the child or others do. Children may reenact traumatic moments by giving directions that are actually scary or upsetting to them to do (or see). Sometimes 'directions' are associated with certain actions (i.e. they may repeat directions they were given during trauma) or be otherwise activating. It is important to be on the lookout for shifts in the child's behavior, mood, attention, or level of involvement—I do not want to inadvertently reinforce overwhelm or dissociation when I am trying for the opposite.

Embodied Body States and Feelings

Communication can be physical. Stories may be told in symptoms and somatic issues, complaints and compulsions (Gaensbauer 2011, Scaer 2014, Silberg 2013, van der Kolk 2014, Wieland 2011). Liam expressed anxiety by becoming hyperfocused on his tummy, and Marcy communicated worry in listless apathy, although neither could initially verbalize what he or she was 'telling.' We need to keep our eyes open to what somatic symptoms, feelings, and behaviors may be representing, so that we can help reframe and normalize children's response to overwhelming situations, help them communicate more clearly, and provide them with healthier alternatives.

Feeding the Insatiable Need: Mika

Mika was adopted from an orphanage overseas at age three. He was five when he started treatment with me for language delay, speech and voice issues, and difficulty chewing. His parents believed that the oral-motor issues were related to the orphanage, where children ate mostly mush. Mika had odd behaviors too, which limited socializing. He ate too fast, grabbed too much, stole food, and hoarded scraps others threw in the garbage. He stashed scraps inside shoes in closets, under his bed, in his book bag, between the headboard and the wall. Mika did not actually eat what he put away. He often forgot where he put food, and could seem genuinely baffled when his parents found a 'cache.' Mika's adoptive mother was sympathetic to his preoccupation with food. She knew that bigger kids often took food from younger ones in the orphanage and that Mika was likely replaying worries he did not have words for. She was less sympathetic, however, to the odors, bugs, and mice.

A year after the adoption, a psychiatrist diagnosed Mika with obsessive-compulsive disorder (OCD) and prescribed medications. These made Mika groggy and ravenous, worsening the hoarding and adding sleepwalking. Undeterred, the doctor recommended locking the fridge and cupboards, but the parents felt that this was wrong to do with a child who had been deprived of food. A family therapist disputed the diagnosis of OCD and informed the parents that this was "about control," recommending they "be firm" and withhold privileges every time "the boy stole food" or "lied about it." Otherwise, he said, they "let him win the battle." To Mika's parents it seemed the battle was not with them but within the child.

I agreed with Mika's parents that his food behaviors were likely clues and communication, and referred them to a therapist with experience with early trauma. Together we set out to help Mika "fill up on" what he missed, working on attachment activities, calming and grounding, narrating routines and verbalizing feelings, recognizing body states, reframing, and regulating. Mika began noting his sensations and we learned that whenever his body was uncomfortable for any reason he experienced "a hole in his tummy" and sought food to make it better. We helped him differentiate sensations, the needs they represented, and the ways to soothe them. As his experience with comfort, regulating, and verbalizing expanded, he was no longer "hungry all over." He recognized he had words to ask for needs to be fulfilled. His food hoarding resolved, but he remained hypersensitive to any hunger pang and frequently complained of "holes stomachaches."

In a stroke of creative genius, Mika's father enrolled him in a cooking class. The boy was delighted! He loved "knowing how to make things to eat" and it provided a sense of control that he would not be helpless around hunger. This turning point freed Mika to attend to other growing. No longer locked into survival, his 'hunger' was satiated and his stomach pains resolved. In spite of residual learning and sensory issues due to deficiencies in infancy and likely prenatal exposures, Mika made excellent progress, flourishing socially in and out of cooking class. He hopes to be a chef when he grows up and teach "other adopted kids how to not be hungry."

Storylines and Narratives

The Story of Everything—Narrating the Seemingly Mundane

Young children enjoy the reassurance of familiarity, and many like listening to the same stories repeatedly. Predictability allows them to internalize the function and structure of stories: a beginning, a middle, and end; characters, actions, and settings; problems, solutions, and resolution (Brinton & Fujiki 1989, Heymann 2010, Ninio & Snow 1996). While they may not have names for these concepts until later childhood, even young children understand and tell stories: the story of going to the park, of spilling juice and cleaning it, of the dog's 'accident' on the carpet. Whether from books or orally, stories combine and integrate experiences into cohesive narrative.

However, narratives may not be so cohesive for traumatized children, who may have less experience with stories, be too activated to process verbal information, or miss parts of the narrative to dissociation. Trauma makes children less available for following events, timelines, causation, sequence, motivation, and logic, ending up with a smattering of disjointed perceptions. Stories are the glue that holds social connections together. When trauma interferes with creating the narrative of what happened and one cannot share what took place, isolation can continue (Cozolino 2006, van der Kolk 2014). Children's story skills are still evolving, which makes them especially vulnerable to the impact of trauma on narrative. Limited narrative also means it is harder to repair or fill in what they cannot explain.

Modeling narrative can provide children with the building blocks for their own narrative. By turning the everyday into stories, we can assist children in understanding and making sense of a world that may feel unpredictable and fragmented. Just as with infants, templates are formed through narrating everyday events. Repetition and scaffolding become the baseline for organizing sensations, causation, sequence, temporal order, impressions, relationships, ideas, and understandings through:

- Telling stories about activities relevant to the child. Talking about events before, during, and after they take place
- Making "story books"—for simple things like 'making breakfast' or 'going to bed,' frequent events like going to the playground, the store, or the zoo, and 'special events' like a birthday party, visiting grandma, or going to the doctor
- Including drawings and/or photos of the child's actions (see below for cautionary note) and people/places/items from the event and accompanying these with narrative offered by you, the child, or the caregiver
- Retelling and revisiting the stories to reinforce familiarity and to incorporate additional emotive language and expanded narrative

- Finding similarities and differences in stories, discussing feelings and sensations (e.g. how your tummy felt before Mommy gave you medicine; how it felt after)
- Highlighting parts of events to tell a story within a story (e.g. at the beach: getting ice cream and Mommy dropping the cone; collecting seashells, finding a beautiful one, and feeling delighted; the dead jellyfish Daddy thought was a plastic bag and jumped back when he realized it wasn't)
- Using books and stories of other people/characters who do similar things as the child, and then adding stories of other times and settings. Literature develops listening and narrative. It allows comparing experience and expands world knowledge and views
- Comparing and contrasting stories to improve observation and description: what was different about Big Bird's visit to the beach? Who did he see, who did you? What did he do, what did you? How did Big Bird feel, how did you? Etc.

Putting in Words without Putting Words In

We often use our own perceptions to infer babies' experiences. Communication is most successful when it is congruent with the baby's experience (e.g. we offer a bottle when the baby is indeed hungry), and familiarity with the baby usually limits misunderstandings and frustration. As children grow they become increasingly able to offer input, and we move to do more elaborating and less guessing. Trauma complicates this process. What we think is taking place may be very different than what traumatized children are actually experiencing or perceiving, yet the children frequently do not know how to correct us.

When we tell stories with children—especially about their own experiences—it is better to offer possibilities rather than statements and make sure that our words make sense to the child. Remaining alert to the child's cues can help us ascertain whether our assumptions are correct so that we can scaffold rather than put words in the child's mouth. For example, a birthday party may not mean happiness and excitement to a maltreated child. It might mean disappointment (if a parent forgot or ignored it) and confusion (if the child had to 'pay up' with sexual favors for his/her presents). It can bring back memories of unpleasant birthdays and worries that bad things would follow. It could awaken grief for someone the child no longer sees.

A car trip to visit Grandma can mean anxiety about being left there or memories of being shuttled between foster placements. Summer vacation might mean worries about hunger (no school lunches), abuse (long weeks at home with maltreating parents), burden (responsibility for younger siblings), jealousy (at what others are doing and the child cannot), and more. Because most maltreatment takes place by people familiar to the child and in everyday settings, we cannot assume that even the most mundane narratives we choose mean the same experience to the child.

Being Tuned to Tenderness—When the Neutral Turns Sensitive

Ricky's father molested her at bedtime. He would "come in to say goodnight" and do things that confused and scared her. It made nighttime routines inherently triggering. Taking a bath, putting on pajamas, brushing teeth, reading a bedtime story—all reminded her of anxieties and the inevitable. Even when her father no longer lived with them, Ricky would get sad and anxious at bedtime. She missed her father. Not his 'yucky' things, but other stuff they did together that was fun. Books made her sad.

For Ricky, the very activity of reading stories was tender: Books reminded her of her father, of all she missed about him and all that scared her. She shut down at school when the teacher read stories, and though she kept asking to be read to at night, she got clingy and fussy. Trauma can make the most basic problematic, and the reality of everyday may not be neutral to the children we see. Dressing, eating, playing, going to the park or school, visiting the doctor, taking a bus, or going for ice cream—no topic is trauma-reminder proof. Keeping aware of shifts in the child's demeanor, affect, engagement, and behavior can clue us to what needs to be handled gently.

A Note about Photos

Photos are increasingly accessible in phones, tablets, and other technology. They make excellent tools for visual cues and mnemonics for events, people, activities, and everyday tasks. Photos can scaffold comprehension, support narrative, and enrich vocabulary. They can be used in story books, sequence and action cards, affect cues, and more. For the majority of children, photos are fun or neutral. Many can be greatly helped by the constancy of photos, which can 'hold' aspects of experiences the child might forget otherwise.

Like everything else trauma touches, photos may not be neutral for some traumatized children. Children who were exploited in child pornography can find the very act of being photographed triggering. Photos can be activating for children whose bruises and injuries were documented for forensics. A child who dissociates may be confused by a photo of something she does not remember because it took place when she was 'spaced out.' Photos can be upsetting for other reasons, too. A child who lost a parent who always took his photograph may feel grief around cameras, and photos of places or certain activities can bring up painful memories or feelings of loss.

I do not avoid photos. In fact, I use them often. However, I rarely take photos of children whose responses I am not familiar with and always begin with taking photos of objects. I ask caregivers to choose (together) some of the child's favorite photos to bring to show me before I ask to or take any new ones of him or her (it also gives me a sense of how the child is with photos). Before I (or their caregiver) take a photo of children, I see if they want to take a photo of me or of something in my office beforehand. I always ask permission to take a photo and pay careful attention to the child's reactions then and at any time photos are presented. Children may say yes not knowing they can say no; they may say yes and then regret it; they may think it feels okay and then it doesn't. I give children a choice whether to take photos home and bring them back or to let me keep the photos between sessions—their photos are theirs to approve and control.

Therapy with traumatized children follows a path similar to other interventions: establishing rapport and building trust, filling in gaps in skills and communication, modeling and scaffolding, practicing and expanding, carrying over to life outside the session. It also requires attention to grounding, connection, attachment, and unmet needs; along with children's sense of safety and their ability to let in support. It calls for awareness to the ways stress and trauma reminders affect children and their ability to attend and learn. Like all therapies, it works best when everyone works together. When collaboration is not possible, we need to optimize the help we are providing while remaining scrupulously within bounds.

16 The Promises and Challenges of Teamwork

Trauma affects multiple aspects of a child's life and development, and traumatized children may need the help of psychologists, speech-language pathologists, occupational and physical therapists, educators, doctors, dentists and orthodontists, hospital staff, and more. The collaboration of caregivers (biological, foster, or adoptive) with child professionals is crucial—so is trauma understanding and open communication among all who work with the child. Otherwise, misconceptions about trauma, institutional red tape, burnout, and denial or dysfunction in caregivers can fragment a child's treatment, becoming barriers to intervention.

Level of Access to Trauma Therapy

The Best—Trauma Therapist Leading the Team

The developmental vulnerability that puts children at high risk for lasting impact of overwhelm also puts them in an excellent position to utilize treatment and remediation. Children's brains are incredibly plastic (Cozolino 2014, Gaensbauer 2011, Schore 2012, Siegel 2012, van der Kolk 2014). Pathways and connections can be 'rewired' to place a child on a healthy (or at least much healthier) developmental trajectory (Levine & Kline 2007, Perry & Szalavitz 2006, Silberg 2013, Wieland 2011). The best scenario for a traumatized child is when a trauma therapist leads the way, sets the pace, and collaborates with other child professionals to ensure that the child is supported in all settings and that everyone is on the same page.

"Hero Book, Please"—Doug Revisited

Doug changed after the car accident that trapped his mom and injured them both (see Chapter 10). Six months later, at age 5:6, Doug's parents brought him to me due to language and processing issues that affected his learning and social behavior. He was aggressive, 'spacey,' and rigid. He'd reportedly had mild language issues before the accident, which worsened since in spite of no sign of brain injury. In addition to speech therapy, Doug's parents sought trauma counseling for the family. The accident left its mark on them, too. "I have nightmares," the mom shared. "He cries for me and I can't help him." The father curtailed work travel, feeling guilty for being away when it happened.

The therapist and I communicated frequently and both of us kept in touch with Doug's kindergarten teachers, who welcomed direction for supporting him. The family worked in psychotherapy to repair the attachment disruption of the accident, while I worked on causation, comprehension, flexibility, and narrative. Doug improved dramatically. Two months into therapy, following several 'stories' of everyday activities, Doug asked to make an 'accident book.' The therapist agreed he was ready. Together we 'wrote' the story of the accident (from which the narrative in Chapter 10 was shaped). It was a tender revisiting, but this time the family was there to provide support for each other, Doug had words for his feelings, and his parents were there to hold him. They met with an ambulance crew and Doug 'explained' to me how they "sometimes give shots to help kids" and that they undress people "to check everywhere" but are "not really mean." Between trauma work with the therapist and language work with me, Doug managed to see the experience as a 'very yucky scary time' that he had gotten through bravely. His parents added to the book, too: his father how he rushed back as fast as he could, his mother how she kept sending him lots of love and hugs even though she had to 'keep still for the firefighters' to get her out of the car safely. Doug named the book, "My Hero Book" and kept asking to read it. He drew a cape on himself in the hospital bed "for being very brave" and stuck gold stars on the paramedic "for helping me" and the police officer "for stopping the cars until Mommy was okay." He added two small figures to the ambulance drawing: "Mom and Dad," he explained soberly, "because they loved me the whole time."

Doug was a well-cared-for child. The collaboration of good trauma therapy and communication work helped reinstate his sense of safety in the world, and words helped him process the experience. His parents were supported as they 'held' his rage and disappointment, confusion and pain, and had space to work through their own helplessness, guilt, and agony. Together, Doug's family integrated the event into a family story and came out stronger for it.

The Good—Available Clinicians Working with Caregivers

Awareness of developmental trauma is growing, but experienced child-trauma therapists are still difficult to find. Even without the lead of a child-trauma therapist, those involved with the family can work together with an open mind—for example, through getting care for the caregivers, who are a child's first line of defense and provide the majority of reparative interactions. Caring for traumatized children means facing difficult realities, challenging behaviors, and strong feelings. Caregivers' issues and buttons are likely to be activated, too.

It is important that they get support and learn how to respond—verbally and otherwise—in ways that scaffold and address the child's needs and reactions.

"Making Up for Lost Time"—Annie Lee Revisited

Annie Lee (see Chapter 5) was adopted from a Chinese orphanage at eighteen months and diagnosed with 'probable autism' a year later. She came to me at two and a half, barely verbal, hardly vocal, still refusing most solids, and showing little interest in symbolic or social play. Her parents worried that she did not know how to love.

Dedicated participants in therapy, Annie Lee's parents learned how to verbalize routines, interpret Annie Lee's communications, and utilize expectation to encourage initiating (e.g. rock and stop so she could indicate more rocking). They provided options (e.g. the red or blue shirt, Mommy's lap or Daddy's); sang and hummed; played peek-a-boo, 'put the toys to sleep,' and 'hide-the-apple.' Uncertain at first, Annie Lee soon showed interest in reciprocity, which became the baseline for auditory attention, discrimination, processing, vocabulary, and comprehension. We took photos and made stories. We clapped and tapped and banged and sang. Feeding work helped her oral-motor skills to mature and support speech-sound production, and vocal play helped her gain better control of her voice. She learned to use her voice to call for others; she realized that she, too, had a name and could be called.

Annie Lee's parents entered therapy to help manage their worries and feelings and to address conflicting views of how to help their daughter. The therapist and I collaborated on practical solutions, and Annie Lee's parents became better at identifying signs of approaching overwhelm and helping her regulate. Everyone got better. After a year of work, the autism diagnosis was firmly off the table. Annie Lee spoke in short sentences, conveying many pragmatic intentions with increasingly intelligible speech. Her play approached age expectations and she blossomed into an affectionate little girl with a contagious giggle. "She's making up for lost time," her mother chuckled.

The 'Just You'—Available Clinician Working Alone

Advances in understanding of trauma, stress, health outcomes, and plasticity should lead to comprehensive prevention and interventions for traumatized children (Cozolino 2014, Gaensbauer 2011, Kendall-Tackett 2002, Scaer 2014, Siegel 2012, Takizawa et al 2014, van der Kolk 2014). In the meanwhile there remain many challenges to care:

- Clinicians who see children at school may have very limited contact with the child's caregivers—paradoxically, especially in areas (e.g. inner-city public schools) where trauma prevalence and caregiver overwhelm are high.
- Schools can have skeletal history, and red tape can make getting more resources difficult, with few 'mandates' (or staff) for counseling or 1:1

therapy. Even when counseling is available, many school psychologists are not trauma trained.

- Disruption of connection can complicate access to care. Many high-risk children (e.g. in foster-care and underprivileged areas) face high turnover and periods without available professional care. One of the hardest realities of working as a consultant for the NYC Department of Education was being in different schools every year. Many of the children I worked with had had too much loss in their short lives already, and I became one more person who 'left.' It broke my heart, especially when I knew that many of them needed all the stability they could get.
- Trauma can be a delicate topic, and clinicians may face active resistance by other child professionals and institutional red tape. Some mental health professionals refuse to consider trauma as part of the child's presentation and insist that other diagnoses and interventions are the way to go (e.g. medications, targeting behaviors without addressing their origins).
- Caregivers may have their own reasons to withhold history or deny the possibility of trauma. Some have preconceived beliefs about the child's difficulties (e.g. autism, bipolar). Feuding parents may have a vested interest in the child's issues, generate additional drama that exacerbates issues, and/or limit access to the child.

Educators, speech-language pathologists, and other child professionals may find themselves the only ones involved in a child's care and need to try and facilitate optimal treatment under less than optimal conditions. Fortunately, even when trauma is not processed directly or teamwork is unavailable, work on grounding, connection, communication, empathy, and stabilization (e.g. see Chapter 14) can help support the child and improve his/her availability to the help offered.

Managing a Less than Optimal Reality

I believe we will soon see much change for the better in the care of developmental trauma. In the meanwhile, each interaction with a child holds potential for repair and offers opportunities for improved grounding, communication, and learning. This is fundamentally important intervention. Also, we can each work to gently involve uninformed and misinformed staff, creatively utilize whatever resources are available, and not be deterred by limited caregiver availability.

Uninformed and Misinformed Staff

My experience has been that when staff are uncooperative it is usually because they are uninformed, misinformed, or burned out. Many professional programs do not teach much about childhood trauma. Textbooks (and popular media) often skim the topic or minimize the impact, especially of sexual abuse and chronic traumatization. Some psychotherapists are intimidated by addressing trauma or worry about forensic and legal issues. Others are 'territorial' and believe that no one outside of mental health should discuss or suggest that trauma needs to be assessed. Clinicians are not above insecurities or denial, and trauma is painful to accept. It is easier to believe that children are not as affected as we know they are; easier to avoid sticky points of discussing maltreatment or loss with caregivers. Many traumatized children do not show signs of overt abuse, and teachers, clinicians, and medical professionals miss or misinterpret signs of overwhelm and have few tools for addressing them. Sometimes those who encounter the most traumatized children inure themselves to the distress by becoming numb themselves.

When staff is unwilling (or unable) to discuss the realities of trauma as possible contributors to the child's issues, I appeal to their greed: How about doing things my way and seeing if it makes their lives easier by improving the child's difficult behaviors? Even skeptical educators tried implementing the tool-kit if it reduced the number of class disruptions and allowed better 'classroom management.' Even skeptical medical personnel tried preparing a child for routine treatment if it made the child less 'high maintenance' to treat. Insensitivity is easy to judge, but caring for traumatized children is difficult and wearying. Many professionals lack sufficient support and can become activated by the children's behaviors and burn out. Acknowledging the challenges they face often opens the door to less confrontational communications, which can then translate into improved collaboration in caring for the child.

Limited Resources

Care costs money, and budgets are often cut in areas that seem like superfluous care. There is strong evidence that adverse childhood events lead to high costs if not attended to (Felitti et al 1998, Kendall-Tackett 2002, Takizawa et al 2014). Yet children in inner-city public schools and foster-care and those with disabilities are still frequently underserved, and many of the children I have worked with had no access to services outside of school. Trauma therapy was often out of the question—their caregivers could not pay—and even if therapy was offered through a community clinic, caregivers could not get the child there if it meant missing work, getting a sitter, or paying travel fares.

Frustrating though lack of care is, creative solutions are worth investigating. Crime-victim clinics may offer therapy for children who witnessed domestic violence. If child therapy is not available, arranging therapy for the parent can often help the child, too. There may be reimbursement for travel, and some community clinics offer child care during caregiver sessions. Volunteers (e.g. big brother/big sister) can add supportive interactions. Presentations for staff and/or residents at women's shelters and for medical and school staff can also increase trauma-aware interactions. Electronic resources can be circulated; books, tapes, and videos borrowed from the library.

Limited Caregiver Support/Availability

Not all traumatized children have caregivers who are involved and motivated. Caregivers' issues may be part of the reason for the child's difficulties. Some care-givers are too occupied with their own issues to help the child or become acti-vated by the child's difficulties, or are logistically unavailable (Evans et al 2006, Haapasalo & Aaltonen 1999, Landy & Menna 2001, Milot et al 2010, O'Shea et al 2000, Sousa et al 2011, Tufnell 2003). When caregivers are uninvolved or under-involved, the challenge for the child increases tenfold. Home is where children are meant to have the most support, and yet it may not be so. Parental discord and distress, homelessness and disability, conflicts of interest, and denial can interfere with a parent's availability to support the child and may even result in derailment of available therapies.

"I Must and I Can't"—Tomas: Parents in the Torment Seat

Tomas was born with a cleft palate and club feet. Reconstructive surgery after birth allowed suckling, but he still had aspirations, pneumonia, and middle-ear infections. He had five surgeries before age two, including muscle flaps to improve palate closure. He had swallowing and feeding issues, unintelligible speech, and limited vocal play and oral exploration. Tomas received speech therapy and physical therapy in early intervention but his "doctor-phobia" and "mouth-phobia" made therapies a struggle.

Tomas was 3:6 when he came to me with speech and language delays. He misbe-haved in school, had short attention span, was easily agitated, and threw "horrible" tantrums. A child psychiatrist diagnosed him with ADHD with possible bipolar disorder. Daily care for Tomas was exhausting: Feeding was a battleground and Tomas had to be restrained for face washing and hair shampooing. He slept poorly, waking multiple times each night.

Tomas' mother feared he would be bullied for his unclear speech and was over-protective, making few age-appropriate demands. She described him as "very sen-sitive," and interventions distressed her. She felt guilty for restraining him as he screamed during doctor visits, and she refused to brush his teeth. "It is like rape and I'm supposed to force it?" she asked in tears. Tomas' father rolled his eyes. He thought his wife overdramatic but admitted feeling overwhelmed when Tomas was born: "He looked like an alien. I felt useless. Couldn't calm him down and he looked scary crying, almost not human." To him Tomas was "spoiled rotten." The par-ents argued about his care at home and during health care appointments, often in Tomas' presence.

Tomas indeed had marked hypersensitivity in his mouth. He avoided tongue movements that touched his palate and could not tolerate anything cold. He indicated moderate pain on a face-pain scale. He had language delays, did not speak much, and instead grabbed what he wanted or pushed things away. He had good understanding of pragmatics but used 'more action, less talk,' in part to compensate for his low intelligibility and in part from impulsivity. His symbolic play was especially aggressive (and expressive). He "put fire" in a lion puppet's mouth, pulled on the tongue, pried it open, and pushed "food" down it "very fast." He covered the puppet's face with a bowl, exclaiming, "Lion bye-bye, lion dead."

I recommended that Tomas' parents meet with a psychotherapist "for support in managing his issues" and in the meanwhile introduced grounding and desensitizing exercises with balls, whistles, bubbles, and straws, along with visualizations, relaxation, and gradual food textures. Tomas' aunt volunteered for home practice, making it fun and conflict free (as long as his parents were not present). Sensitivity in Tomas' mouth normalized dramatically, with better feeding tolerance, increased intelligibility, and more communicative success. Being understood helped Tomas socially and behaviorally.

He remained, however, "exceedingly difficult" at home. The parents decided against family therapy, going instead to a behavioral child therapist, who stated that Tomas' "controlling" behavior in the present was the issue, not "things from infancy." Battles over meals and daily care escalated. Mom refused to "force" Tomas, while Dad demanded too much and resented being made the 'bad guy.' Fights and strain led to divorce, with Tomas living mostly with his mother, who stopped therapies and enrolled him in special education with diagnoses of ADHD and sensory integration disorder.

Unaddressed, the distress both parents and child endured continued to be communicated through conflict even after Tomas' skills improved. His mother was frightened, his father could be frightening; both were overwhelmed. Tomas was furious and terrified and the trauma continued to be expressed and reinforced by daily conflicts and relational drama. Tomas' parents loved him, but I believe their own issues got in the way of his care, creating endless feedback loops of double-binds.

Bias and Overmedicating

With insurance companies that aim for quick fixes, pharmaceutical companies that promote medications, and the distressing realties of childhood trauma, one can see how children with trauma presentations may more readily get diagnosed with attention-deficit hyperactivity disorder (ADHD), autism, bipolar disorder, etc. As discussed in Chapter 12, these are valid diagnoses for some children. Also, medications certainly have their place and can help some children manage till their systems are better regulated. However, all too often children are diagnosed without taking trauma into account, medicated instead of treated, and have trauma reactions and communications of distress smothered under escalated doses (Silberg 2013, Waters 2005, Wieland 2011). Some could be due to lack of awareness of developmental trauma and its presentation and some due to differing views about what certain behaviors indicate and how to treat them (Beitchman et al 1996, Carey 2007, Christian 2008, Danon-Boileau 2002, Kearney 2006, Schwartz 2013, 2014). For example, if distractibility in a child is seen to indicate ADHD, one may not see hypervigilance.

It can be easier for caregivers to accept nontrauma diagnoses, too. It is understandable. Trauma implies something that happened to the child and might have been prevented, rather than something one was born with. Chronic trauma, maltreatment, or attachment disruption implies that someone's actions or inaction played a role in the child's distress and may require the adults to change in order for the child to heal—something some caregivers are not ready to face or do. Yet a million cases of maltreatment are substantiated in the US alone annually, with over 90% of maltreatment by people close to the child (US-DHHS 2013a): We likely all know some children who have been harmed by loved ones. Other traumas are difficult to accept, too: that a child was traumatized by the very actions done to save her, that a mother's postpartum depression caused neglect, that an addiction exacted a lasting price. People go to great lengths to avoid guilt and shame (Freyd & Birrell 2013, Howell 2011, Shaw et al 2006, van der Hart et al 2006) and trauma realities can be painful. Even when trauma does not imply culpability, professionals can be reluctant to mention it lest they be seen as 'blaming' and lead to the parent withdrawing the child from treatment altogether.

I rarely challenge a child's psychiatric diagnosis, especially not before I know the child well, and/or if clinicians are not open to considering the impact of overwhelm. However, I may raise the possibility of comorbidity and offer alternative explanations for some of the child's behaviors, along with some solutions to minimize them. When trauma history is known, I often mention trauma's impact on regulation, attention, and processing and offer suggestions for working on those. Very often, symptoms improve and medication is scaled back with overall benefits to the child.

Ongoing Stress and Retraumatization

What do we do when a traumatized child continues to experience overwhelm? How do we help a child be less flooded when life continues to be traumatizing? How can children learn to feel safe when they are not really safe yet? How can they be present when they still need to take themselves away? Unfortunately this is reality for children with ongoing homelessness, custody and foster-care placements, continued medical challenges, and all manner of war zones.

For these children, safety may be only relative. Connection may be temporary. Attachment may be tentative. Being present may be limited to certain settings, people, and times. Limitations do not make opportunities for grounding and compassion any less real or important. If nothing else, respite moments can be all the more crucial if only for establishing that there is something beyond overwhelm: that calm and care are possible, that learning can offer a different kind of an escape, that words can bridge some of the gulfs trauma forms.

We may not be able to remove the trauma from some children's lives or provide the room for them to process it, but we can still make space for being present, for narrating states and emotions, and for clarifying how some things lead to others (even if much else in life boggles comprehension). Longitudinal study of traumatized children in Israel found that sometimes the difference between children who do better and those who do not can be the presence of an adult in their lives who provided reparative experiences (Zimrin 1986). Our interventions may be brief and limited, but we never know if they may become an anchor for hope.

The Crucial Importance of Remaining within Bounds

I have lost count of times I wanted to take children home with me and make it all better. Bringing clients home to mother them to health is not going to cut it in the boundaries department ... but it is information. This feeling is a compass: It only happens when I feel protective, whether I know why or not. It usually signals a child in distress or need and tells me to keep very clear about what I can or cannot do while remaining within my scope of practice.

The Difference between Responding to Trauma and Processing Trauma

Responding to children's distress and ensuring their safety is every adult's responsibility. Helping children regulate, maintaining safe boundaries, and offering support are the responsibility of all child professionals. As a speech-language pathologist, these responsibilities extend to offering reciprocity, providing context, modeling narrative and interaction, scaffolding communication, ensuring comprehension, facilitating processing, verbalizing causation and expectation, formulating and responding to questions, identifying and repairing miscommunications, and supporting social language, among other tasks. It includes recognizing shifts in a child's relating and responding to them. Providing tools to process the world with is my job. Direct trauma processing is not. Teaching emotive language is my job. Inquiring about the experience of a trauma is not. Verbalizing and elaborating on what a child brings up spontaneously is my job. Asking about the minutiae of traumatic events is not.

Speech-language pathologists help children build foundations from which they can venture into the world to communicate with others and verbalize both internal and external experiences to themselves and to those around them. We model how communication works and provide children opportunities to master it. We help children get to where they can understand, process, and relate with others; and we can hope that these tools will stand them in good stead when they need to address life in joy as well as challenge.

"This One's Okay"—Marcus Revisited

Marcus (see Chapter 8) was terrorized by his great-aunt and would shut down around any printed matter. Reading and being read to were too much, but his every-day was filled with such demands. Marcus was eight. The coping skills that got him through an intolerable past were strangling his present. His mother agreed to place him on a waiting list for a local community mental health clinic. In the meanwhile we had to help him manage the trigger without delving into the trauma that distorted it. I changed Marcus' sessions to the class's reading time—to limit his need to dissociate and allow him use of that time for working with me on stabilization and language support.

An upcoming field trip to the Museum of Natural History became an opportunity. Marcus loved animals and was very excited about the excursion. I asked him what he hoped to see and gave him index cards to draw elephants, the whale, tigers, dinosaur-bones, Native American things. While he did that, I used other index cards and wrote what he knew and/or wanted to find out about each. We took the cards to the museum and "checked" for answers on the plaques. I gave Marcus my camera to take photos of exhibits he found interesting. We reviewed the photos the following session as I "took notes" and added index cards with his impressions.

"How long did mammoth tusks get?" Marcus asked suddenly.

"Hmm, that's a great question. Where do you think we can find out?"

He gave me a wary look. Children know when you ask a question you already have the answer for. "The Internet?" he tried. I typed the question in and read to him what we found. His eyes grew huge with wonder when we measured 16 feet in the hallway. "Maybe add it to the mammoth card," I offered. Marcus did not hesitate, rifling through the cards for the "Wooly Mammoth" and copying the detail in.

The next session, I taped the cards with his drawings, those with queries, the corresponding photos, and the 'notes' onto sheets of paper. "Should we staple them together?" I offered, holding the collated pages.

"You're making a book." His voice was accusatory. He looked scared.

"Not all books are scary, Marcus," I said gently. "You are safe here and these are all pages we put together ourselves. There is no scary stuff here."

He nodded.

"We don't have to staple the pages, but it will help keep them from getting lost."

"Can we put a paper-clip?" he asked. We did. Flipping through the pages, I read to him what was already there and we added more things he recalled.

"It's kind of a book," he noted in half-query/half-challenge.

"Yes, kind of a book about the story of our visit to the museum," I added. "A really good story, too." He paused.

"Not all stories are bad or scary, Marcus," I repeated. "I don't like scary books or stories, either. But I like learning new and interesting things that are not scary. This kind of a book we made together is an interesting and a very safe story, a not-scary book."

Marcus took a breath and looked at me searchingly. "I don't like books," he said quietly.

"I know," I replied gently. "I'm sorry."

He held my eyes then looked back at the stack of papers on the desk. "This one's okay, though," he added, "maybe we should staple them so they don't get messed up . . ."

Marcus' wariness around books and stories did not disappear that day, but he stayed present through the realization of what this was and it helped him see how it was safely different. He continued to build more tolerance for managing printed matter without dissociating, as over the next sessions we wrote more notes and made a cardboard cover for his museum book. He proudly wrote "Great stuff at the Museum, By Marcus" on it, and the teacher's praise had him glowing. He let her read it to the class, then took the book home to read with his mother. We collated other 'books' about whales and dolphins and visited the school library together—a big step for a boy who would shut down upon entry—to borrow some books for the project. Marcus was learning: Not all stories were scary. Not all books were bad. Not all questions were tricky. It was safe to listen and worth it to know how to read to find out all the stuff there was to know about.

My work with Marcus was in some way desensitization, though it was done as any speech-language work would be done—small steps the child could manage toward long-term goals of improved listening comprehension, reading comprehension, and expressive writing. I never pried about why he found books and stories scary. It would have been okay if he chose to share what scared him or anything about what he had gone through and I would have offered grounding and general support if he had. However, as a rule I do not probe for trauma details myself. It may seem a fine line between support and inquiry, but keeping communication and validation as the goals keeps the boundary clear: My role is not to process the trauma itself but to help the child feel safer in the present and give him tools to process life—and trauma—in their appropriate settings.

The Stages of Trauma Therapy—Who Should Do What, When, and How

As understanding of trauma grew over the last few decades, therapy guidelines have been established for both adults and children. These guidelines follow three general stages, with work cycling between stages throughout intervention (van der Hart et al 2006, ISSTD 2004, 2011, Loewenstein 2006, Wieland 2011):

Stage One—Stabilization and symptom reduction: The main goals are to establish safety and build attachment, set safe limits, develop skills for calming and grounding, and introduce psychoeducation about the effects of trauma (for the child, caregivers, and other adults in the child's life). Building the child's attachment with the parent/caregiver is best, though at times attachment to the therapist is necessary (e.g. when caregivers are not actively engaged in the therapy). This stage is applicable to any clinician working with traumatized children. It includes awareness of trauma reactions; addressing distorted beliefs and misconceptions about self, people, and the world; and helping the child get grounded and present enough to reconnect with his/her body and experiences. Stage One work provides a foundation for regulation and verbalization, awareness and safety, and is well within the scope of practice of speech-language pathologists and other child professionals. When collaborative work is not possible, clinicians should offer stabilization, validate a child's experience, and reduce overwhelm. They should also take care to not dismantle defenses the child still needs: Until children can work through their trauma, they may need to apply dissociation when they get overwhelmed.

Stage Two—Trauma processing: In this stage, a psychotherapist works with the child on dealing directly with the trauma through addressing the fragmented memories of trauma and managing and processing dissociated feelings. This stage should be done by a trauma therapist skilled in titrating overwhelm and addressing dissociation and is not part of the work that speech-language pathologists do. As with Marcus, general support is appropriate, but direct exploration of trauma and dismantling dissociative barriers should not be done outside of trauma therapy. When collaborative treatment is available, child professionals will be advised that the child is processing trauma so they understand possible escalation/changes and continue to provide supportive (i.e. Stage One) work while the psychotherapist addresses the trauma with the child and caregivers.

Stage Three—Integration and learning new coping skills: In this stage, work expands to include skills for managing ongoing stress and healthy reactions to possible overwhelm. It also involves addressing skills that lagged behind. In collaborative therapy, the speech-language pathologist and other child professionals can assist in closing gaps and reinforcing better life skills in the child.

'Rescuer,' 'Fixer,' and the Reality of 'Good Enough'

Clinicians enter the healing professions to help others. We want to make it all better. When that is impossible—especially when it comes to children—it is heartbreaking. It may also become a recipe for boundary breaching: taking on more than we can do, promising more than we can give, delving beyond scope of practice, taking on the role of parents when we cannot be that for the child. It shattered me to know that children went home to less-than-good-enough, that they were lonely and possibly scared, that they would once again be shuttled between homes, witness violence, endure pain. I wanted to shelter them, fix everything that was broken, and heal them so the heartbreak they endured would be no more. Wanting to rescue children is normal. It is important: Whenever I suspected a child was in danger, I made the call to those who could investigate and did what I could in support. However, I could not prevent all harm or hardship. Knowing it and taking care so I can stay plugged in anyway is maybe the most important thing I can do—along with loving the children, caring about them, being kind and gentle, offering the best therapeutic interaction I can manage, teaching skills for verbalizing life, modeling, and providing the tools for a different experience. This is rarely all that's needed, but at times it can be—must be—'good enough.'

17 Supporting the Supporters

Recognizing and Managing Secondary Traumatization

Vicarious (Secondary) Traumatization and 'Burnout'

Secondary traumatization happens when the trauma of other persons overwhelms those who care for them (Figley 1995, Pearlman & Saakvitne 1995). It is a common occupational hazard for professionals working with traumatized children (6%–26% of child therapists, up to 50% of caseworkers), and some symptoms of secondary traumatization include: hypervigilance, hopelessness, guilt, avoidance, minimizing, cynicism, sleeplessness, withdrawal, insensitivity to violence, anger, illness, fear, chronic exhaustion, poor boundaries, reduced self-care, and loss of creativity and zest for life (Rothchild 2006, Saakvitne & Pearlman 1996). Rather than a sign of weakness, any of these is often due to compassion and empathy. Any professional working directly with trauma is at risk, but more so those individuals who are highly empathetic (or who have their own unresolved trauma—see following segment), those who have a heavy caseload of trauma clients, and/or who feel isolated or inadequately trained. Whenever secondary traumatization symptoms appear, it is important to attend to them: Secondary traumatization can lead to shutting down, 'burnout' and leaving the field, and/or loss of trust in the safety of the world we live in (Mathieu 2011, Rothchild 2006).

When surrounded by children who have been hurt, it is understandable to begin to feel as if harm is everywhere. However, clinicians already see a skewed population: The children who come to see us are by definition struggling and represent a high-risk section of the population. It helps to remember that most children are not harmed, that many adults make 'good enough' caregivers, that not all medical intervention is traumatizing to children, that most children are not terribly neglected, and most brief attachment disruptions get repaired without lasting impact. While this does not trivialize the numbers of traumatized children or makes any level of maltreatment acceptable, it can help preserve our perspective of the world and society.

Seek support if you have:

- Intrusive thoughts (e.g. obsessing over whether anyone hurt your healthy child; seeing every tantrum or 'silent treatment' as a 'sure sign' of trauma;

finding it difficult to be intimate because of thoughts of children's sexual abuse)
- Anxiety and overprotectiveness of children
- Guilt (e.g. for having a safe house or healthy children, for eating good food when some do not have it)
- Suspicion and distrust without cause (e.g. distrusting all agencies or case-workers, believing you need to do everything yourself—including crossing boundaries—because no one else will 'save the children')
- Helplessness and despair (e.g. feeling like no matter what you do, nothing is enough, the world is mean, people are cruel, and it is best to not bring children into the world)
- Apathy and 'being inured' to children's distress, feeling numb
- Difficulty concentrating, loss of focus, feeling deskilled, frequent second-guessing
- Feeling burned out, skipping work, contemplating quitting
- Difficulty sleeping

When the Clinician's Past Awakens

Childhood trauma has been a reality for generations, but attention to it is relatively recent. This means that many adults who endured childhood traumas never got help for it. In some people, childhood overwhelm did not become disruptive in clearly identifiable ways, while in others it may have manifested in fears, depression, anxiety, addictions, difficulties with intimacy and relationships, underachieving, health issues, and more (Danese et al 2009, Felitti et al 1998, Ferguson & Dacey 1997, Kendall-Tackett 2002, Scaer 2014, Takizawa et al 2014). Clinicians and educators are not exempt from having had childhood challenges. In fact many who go into the helping professions do so because they understand children's agony and want to alleviate it (Figley 1995, Rothchild 2006). While not every child professional survived childhood trauma, for some of us being exposed to children's pain may awaken our own experience of overwhelm.

Children's distress can be triggering. Adults who witnessed domestic violence can find an out-of-control child a reminder of others who blew their gasket. A frightened child may trigger a memory of oneself cowering. A medically vulnerable child may trigger the complex feelings one had for ill siblings or parents, or memories of one's own medical confusion and overwhelm. When we bring ourselves to the interaction, we are bound to have all manner of things awaken in us: compassion, protectiveness, care, affection, kindness, joy, and pride, along with worry, helplessness, despair, confusion, frustration, and pains of our past (Figley 1995, Pearlman & Saakvitne 1995, Rothchild 2006, Wallin 2007).

There need be no shame in having one's own trauma pay a visit. Just as in the children, our bodies too can react to reminders of time passed (Scaer 2014, van der Kolk 2014). What is important is to recognize such activation and seek support for it. It is never too late to process life's overwhelm: We should do so for ourselves, for others in our lives who otherwise will bear the brunt of our own activation, for the children we want to keep helping. If your history rears its head, get support. You deserve it. It is worth it. You are worth it.

Attachment Wounds and Old Tapes

Not all things that get triggered are identifiable traumas. Some activate a more sneaky kind of repeating: attachment wounds and 'old tapes' that replay what we have internalized and causes pain. Reaction to interaction is normal—if we did not react, we would not be engaged. Some people 'bring out the best in us,' others, not so much. Children are not exempt from activating adults in both comfortable and uncomfortable ways. There are children with whom it feels rewarding to interact; children we feel comfortable with, accepted and appreciated by. Then there are those children who 'push our buttons' and whose sessions we may come to dread. A rise in blood pressure in reaction to an 'obstinate' preschooler is a disproportionate reaction to the muscle-flexing of a little one testing his or her control. Rather, the child may be activating one's own rage at someone—maybe a parent—who discounted needs or ignored requests or calls for help. A child who lashes out with "I hate you," "you are mean," "you suck" can activate one's old tapes of feeling unloved and misunderstood by others who were dismissive or unkind.

Activation is information: pause-buttons to let us know that something is being replayed and amplified which is not about the child but may well be about old wounds and relating patterns we need to attend to (Pearlman & Saakvitne 1995). It is a form of 'counter-transference'—par for the course in clinical involvement—worthy of seeking support through self-reflection, peer consultation, and/or supervision. Awareness of our own activation is a clinical asset that can deepen our own growth and make us more fully available to those we seek to support. Not addressing it risks our own attachment issues interfering with our ability to identify, comprehend, and attend to the child's needs.

Disillusion and Perceived Helplessness

Many of us work in less than optimal conditions with less than optimal resources. It can be heartbreaking to know that children in dire needs fall through the cracks or are not getting the right therapies, do not have 'good enough' caregivers, lack stability and safety. It might feel like the small adjustments we can make cannot possibly ameliorate the stresses and awfulness children meet daily. Red tape, lack of awareness, minimization, refusing to allocate resources, organizational denial, case-worker inaccessibility, caregiver apathy—can lead to disillusionment about the ability to help the children in any meaningful way.

In some way, disillusion and helplessness mirror the child's experience. The realities we find ourselves in while trying to assist the children hold some of the same emotions children manage: despair, frustration, distrust, helplessness, hopelessness. We may be picking up on their despair as they communicate if not in words then in affect. I have found it helpful to take a step back from the child's reality to reevaluate the present, which may well be frustrating but maybe not desperate. Someplace in all the 'cannot,' I try to identify some 'can do.'

When I first worked in inner-city public schools, I often felt disillusioned. My sister, Dr. Ruth Rosen-Zvi, a clinical child psychologist and trauma expert in Israel, taught me that even what I see as very limited still matters. "Would you take that away from them, too?" she asked, and shared how even one adult providing a reparative experience can make the difference (Zimrin 1986). It was not about 'good' but about doing 'the best good enough.' I realized that even if all I managed to do was allow children to recognize 'safer' and believe that they were worthy of care, it mattered. My wish to 'save the kids' could be funneled into doing my best: to arrange for more care, a better classroom, compassion from teachers so they do not see the children as menaces but more as children in need.

Sometimes there is little we can do to affect visible change in a child's life. Many children deserve better than the care they are getting, while all too many people in power remain ignorant of trauma and the need to address it. It is natural to feel frazzled by stalled systems, numbing paperwork, apathy, and denial. Nonetheless we can offer reparative exchanges, model care, and kindness, and 'hear' what the child is communicating. Addressing what we can matters, even if only within the limited settings of our interactions with the children. As long as we remain plugged in, we are not helpless to create change. Every interaction is potential. Don't let frustration immobilize you. Be the best clinician you can be for those who come your way; reach out and educate; volunteer with organizations that work to improve understanding of developmental trauma and access to therapies. Change can happen with each one of us and together we can reduce helplessness and overwhelm.

Finding a Professional 'Home'

A good way to mitigate frustration, minimize secondary trauma, and feel supported is by becoming part of professional organizations that deal with trauma and dissociation. It helps to share our experiences with like-minded individuals who 'get' us and understand what we do and why we do it. Organizations like the ISSTD—the International Society for the Study of Trauma and Dissociation— offer a professional home to clinicians, academics, researchers, health workers, legal personnel, students, emerging professionals, and educators who work with traumatized children, teens, and adults (www.isst-d.org). Annual conferences, regional workshops, online seminars, listservs, and peer groups can provide opportunities for professional growth, widening skill sets, venting, brainstorming, and collegial connections and friendships. The National Child Traumatic Stress Network (NCTSN), the Institute on Violence, Abuse, and Trauma (IVAT), and other organizations carry information and resources. You do not need to go it alone.

Making Time to Play, Laugh, Love, and Rest

Health requires balance. Time to work, time to play; time to be serious, time to be silly; time to rest; time to love; time to laugh. It all sounds lovely on paper but child professionals often find themselves overworking and underplaying. There is just so much to do. . . . We may feel compelled to take on too many cases because there is no one to refer to; feel unable to find time for something as trivial as meeting a friend; struggle to take vacations when these destabilize some clients; feel the need to be the one reliable adult these children (and sometimes their caregivers) have and so become available 24/7. I have certainly been guilty of all the above and still feel this way frequently. It comes with the territory. Like many caretakers, I am an overprotective certifiable mother-hen. What I had to learn was that my level of self-care is in direct proportion to my ability to be there for my clients, and that having the above worries usually signaled my having lapsed on rest and play.

The metaphor of keeping our own cup full is true here. We cannot offer someone a drink from a bone-dry cup and cannot be supportive if we have nothing to give. This lesson in self-care is even more important when we aim to provide a model for identifying, verbalizing, responding, and regulating body states and needs. If we do not attend to our needs, what are we teaching the children who come to us not knowing how to identify or respond to their own? If we do not make time for relationships, what model are we providing a child who does not know how to form or keep friendships? Just as we would like for our clients, we need to mindfully make time and free up energy for laughter, playfulness, exploration, creativity, curiosity, friendships, love, and intimacy.

Considering Counseling

Taking care of traumatized children is not simple or neutral. For some of us, it can awaken old wounds or bring closer times we prefer to have forgotten. It can press tender points and activate old tapes, beliefs, or memories. Stoicism and empathy do not mix well. We would not ask the children we work with to put on a stiff upper lip and go on as if nothing happened, and we should not demand this of ourselves. Resilience does not mean ignoring or pretending pain is not there but is the strength born of facing, knowing, processing, and growing beyond it.

Taking care of ourselves is important not only for us, but for our clients. We may need a place to process our own reactions and realities, our pains and wounding, our biases and worries, the things that clients activate in us, the unworded and untold feelings and realities in ourselves. Sometimes a close trusted friend, spouse, partner, clergy, or peer group offers that support. However, for many of us who work with traumatized youngsters, seeking individual counseling can be a good way to attend to our own needs and history. Some clinicians attend therapy or supervision on an as-needed basis when issues arise. Others prefer ongoing therapy and use it to process both past pain and current challenges—especially when a history of childhood trauma may become activated (in aware and not-so-aware ways) by children in one's care. A friend used to say: "All the martyrs are dead, so aiming to become a martyr is a darn fool way to live . . . " There are different paths to self-care, and our own needs are as worthy as those of others. Like the children, we too do our best work when we are well cared for.

Afterword
A Prognosis of Hope

There is healing from trauma. There is language after silence and connection after the loneliness of overwhelm. While no amount of care will prevent all pain from happening, and as long as there are bad neighborhoods, bad schools, poverty, and war, limiting realities will exist; still much can be repaired. One thing we can all do is increase understanding of trauma in children and adolescents—not just because we know its costs, but because we know that years of suffering can be spared and amazing growth be gained.

Speech-language pathologists I worked with unanimously wished that developmental trauma and its implications on communication had been part of the curriculum in their programs and professional development. I found the same in teachers, dentists, nurses, pediatricians, psychologists, social workers, foster-parents, and adoptive parents. It makes sense: We all see these children. Of course trauma affects them. Trauma and dissociation are not limited to psychotherapy offices, and communication difficulties are not segregated to speech-language pathologists' offices or special education classes. Medical, behavioral, developmental, and relational issues affect children wherever they are. Let's make trauma and how it affects communication part of every child-profession program, so we all know what we are seeing and can collaborate to support traumatized children and teens. Together, we can keep a porch light on for hope.

"I think that maybe I'm going to be okay." (G., age 13)

"I used to be sad everywhere inside me but now I have words to tell things, and my feelings are more glad." (Leila, age 7)

"Did you know bodies can be tingly? My leg fell asleep so I grounded it." (M., age 8)

"It's all better in my heart now." (Doug, age 5)

"My favorite word is 'I love you,' oh and 'ice-cream.'" (Annie Lee, age 4)

"I called Mommy and Mommy came." (Manuel, age 2:6)

References

Adams, J. A. (1994). *Beginning to Read: Thinking and Learning about Print,* Cambridge, MA, MIT Press.

Albers, L., Barnett, E. D., Jenista, J. A., Johnson, D. E. (Eds) (2005). International adoption: Medical and developmental issues, *Pediatric Clinics of North America,* 53(5):13–15.

Anand, K. J., Hickey, P. R. (1987). Pain and its effects in the human neonate and fetus, *New England Journal of Medicine,* 317(21):1321–1329.

Attias, R., Goodwin, J. (1999). *Splintered Reflections: Images of the Body in Trauma,* New York: Basic Books.

Balsamo, L. M., Benjamin, X., Grandin, C. B., Petrella, J. R., Braniecki, S. H., et al (2008). A functional magnetic resonance imaging study of left hemisphere language dominance in children, *Journal of Neuroscience,* 28(47):12176–12182.

Barakat, L. P., Kazak, A. E., Gallagher, P. R., Meeske, K., Stuber, M. (2000). Posttraumatic stress symptoms and stressful life events predict the long-term adjustment of survivors of childhood cancer and their mothers, *Journal of Clinical Psychology in Medical Settings,* 7(4):189–196.

Baron, N. S. (1992). *Growing Up with Language: How Children Learn to Talk,* Reading, MA: Addison-Wesley.

Barth, E. P., Freundlich, M., Brodzinsky, D. (Eds) (2000). *Adoption & Prenatal Alcohol and Drug Exposure: Research, Policy, and Practice,* Washington DC: Child Welfare League of America.

Beitchman, J. H., Cohen, N., Konstantareas, M. M., Tannock, R. (1996). *Language, Learning, And Behavior Disorders: Developmental, Biological, And Clinical Perspectives,* Cambridge: Cambridge University Press.

Bell, N. J., McGhee, P. E., Duffey, N. S. (1986). Interpersonal competence, social assertiveness and the development of humour, *British Journal of Developmental Psychology,* 4:51–55.

Bellis, T. J. (2002). *When the Brain Can't Hear: Unraveling the Mystery of Auditory Processing Disorder,* New York: Pocket Books.

Benedict, M. I., White, R. B., Wulff, L. M., Hall, B. J. (1990). Reported maltreatment of children with multiple disabilities, *Child Abuse & Neglect,* 14: 207–217.

Bennett, D. S., Wolan Sullivan, M., Lewis, M. (2010). Neglected children, shame-proneness, and depressive symptoms, *Child Maltreatment* 15:305.

Berman, R. (Ed.) (2004). *Language Development across Childhood and Adolescence,* Philadelphia: John Benjamins.

Beverly, B., McGuinness, T., Blanton, D. (2008). Communication challenges for children adopted from the former Soviet Union, *Language, Speech, and Hearing Services in Schools,* 39: 1–11.

Bialystok, E. (2001). *Bilingualism in Development: Language, Literacy, and Cognition*, Cambridge: Cambridge University Press.

Blanc, R. Adrien, J. L., Roux, S., Barthélémy, C. (2005). Dysregulation of pretend play and communication development in children with autism, *Autism*, 9:229.

Bowlby, J. (1997). *Attachment and Loss, Vol. 1*. London: Random House.

Bremmer, J. D., Randall, P., Vermetten, E., Staib, L. Bronen, R., et al (1997). Magnetic resonance imaging-based measurement of hippocampal volume in posttraumatic stress disorder related to childhood physical and sexual abuse—a preliminary report, *Biological Psychiatry*, 41(1):23–32.

Brewin, C. (2005). Encoding and retrieval of traumatic memories. In J. Vasterling & C. Brewin (Eds) *PTSD: Biological, Cognitive, and Clinical Perspectives* (pp. 131–135). New York: Guilford Press.

Brinton, B., Fujiki, M. (1989). *Conversational Management with Language-Impaired Children: Pragmatic Assessment and Intervention*, Excellence in Practice Series, Katharine C. Butler, Editor, Aspen Publishers, Inc.

Briscoe-Smith, A. M., Hinshaw, S. P. (2006). Linkages between child abuse and attention-deficit/hyperactivity disorder in girls: Behavioral and social correlates, *Child Abuse and Neglect*, 30(11):1239–1255.

Browne, J. V. (2003). New perspectives on premature infants and their parents, *Zero to Three*, November:1–12.

Bruning, P. A. (2007). The crisis of adoption disruption and dissolution. In N. Boyd Webb (Ed), *Play Therapy with Children in Crisis*, 3rd ed: *Individual, Group, and Family Treatment*, New York: Guilford Press.

Bryant, B., Mayou, R., Wiggs, L., Ehlers, A., Stores, G. (2004). Psychological consequences of road traffic accidents for children and their mothers, *Psychological Medicine*, 34:335–346.

Bryden, M. P., Munhall, K., Allard, F. (1983). Attentional biases and the right-ear effect in dichotic listening, *Brain and Language*, 18(2):236–248.

Cappadocia, M. C., Weiss, J. A., Pepler, D. (2011). Bullying experiences among children and youth with autism spectrum disorder, *Journal of Autism and Developmental Disorders*, 42(2):266–277.

Carbajal, R., Rousset, A., Danan, C., Coquery, S., Nolent, P., et al (2008). Epidemiology and treatment of painful procedures in neonates in intensive care units, *Caring for the Critically Ill Patient: JAMA*, 300(1):60–70.

Carey, B. (2007). Bipolar illness soars as a diagnosis for the young, *New York Times*, September 4, 2007.

Carlsson, A. A., Kihlgren, A., Sørlie, S. (2008). Embodied suffering: Experiences of fear in adolescent girls with cancer, *Journal of Child Health Care*, 12:129.

Carter, B. (2002). Chronic pain in childhood and the medical encounter: Professional ventriloquism and hidden voices, *Qualitative Health Research*, 12:28.

Casey, F. A., Sykes, D. H., Craig, B. G., Power, R., Mulholland, H. C. (1996). Behavioural adjustment of children with complex congenital heart disease, *Journal of Pediatric Psychology*, 21:335–352.

Choe, M., Ortiz-Mantilla, S., Makris, N., Gregas, M., Bacic, J., et al (2013). Regional infant brain development: An MRI-based morphometric analysis in 3 to 13 month olds, *Cerebral Cortex*, 23(9):2100–2117.

Christian, C. (2008). Professional education in child abuse and neglect, *Pediatrics*, 122:S13–S17.

Cohen, N. J. (2001). *Language Impairment and Psychopathology in Infants, Children, and Adolescents*, Developmental Clinical Psychology and Psychiatry series, Vol. 45, Thousand Oaks, CA: Sage Publications.

Cole, S. F., O'Brien, J. G., Gadd, G., Ristuccia, J., Wallace, L., Gregory, M. (2005). *Helping Traumatized Children Learn: Supportive School Environments for Children Traumatized by Family Violence.* Boston: Advocates For Children.

Cournos, F. (1999). *City of One: A Memoir,* New York: Plume Publishing, the Penguin Group.

Cozolino, L. (2006). *The Neuroscience of Human Relationships: Attachment and the Developing Brain,* New York: Norton.

Cozolino, L. (2014). *The Neuroscience of Human Relationships: Attachment and the Developing Social Brain,* 2nd ed, Norton Series on Interpersonal Neurobiology, New York: W. W. Norton And Company.

Cross, M. (2004). *Children with Emotional and Behavioural Difficulties and Communication Problems: There Is Always a Reason.* London: Jessica Kingsley Publishers.

Crosse, S., Elyse, K., Ratnofsky, A. (1993). *A Report on the Maltreatment of Children with Disabilities.* Washington, DC: National Center On Child Abuse And Neglect, U.S. Department of Health and Human Services.

Danese, A., Moffitt, T. E., Harrington, H. L., Milne, B. J., Polanczyk, G., et al (2009). Adverse childhood experiences and adult risk factors for age-related disease: Depression, inflammation, and clustering of metabolic risk markers, *Archives of Pediatric and Adolescent Medicine,* 163(12):1135–1143.

Danon-Boileau, L. (2002). *Children without Language: From Dysphasia to Autism,* New York: Oxford University Press.

Davison, M. D., Hammer, C., Lawrence, F. R. (2011), Associations between preschool language and first grade reading outcomes in bilingual children, *Journal of Communication Disorders,* 44(4):444–458.

Daud, A., Skoglund, E., Rydelius, P.-A. (2005). Children in families of torture victims: Transgenerational transmission of parents' traumatic experiences to their children, *International Journal of Social Welfare,* 14:23–32.

Deater-Deckard, K. (2005). Parenting stress and children's development: Introduction to the special issue, *Infant and Child Development,* 14:111–115.

De Bellis, M. D. (2005). The psychobiology of neglect, *Child Maltreatment,* 10(2):150–172.

de Boysson-Bardies, B. (1999). *How Language Comes to Children: From Birth to Two Years,* Boston: MIT Press.

Decety, J., Chaminate, T., Grezes, J., Meltzoff, A. N. (2002). A PET exploration of the neural mechanisms involved in reciprocal imitation, *Neuroimage,* 15 (1):265–272.

Decety, J., Chaminade, T. (2003). When the self represents the other: A new cognitive neuroscience view on psychological identification, *Consciousness and Cognition.* 12:577–596.

Degangi, G. A., Kendall, A. (2008). *Effective Parenting for the Hard-to-Manage Child: A Skills-Based Book,* New York: Routledge, Taylor & Francis Group.

Dell'Api, M., Rennick, J. E., Rosmus, C. (2007). Childhood chronic pain and health care professional interactions: Shaping the chronic pain experiences of children, *Journal of Child Health Care,* 11:269.

Denham, S. A. (1998). *Emotional Development in Young Children.* New York: Guilford Press.

Diseth, T. H. (2006). Dissociation following traumatic medical treatment procedures in childhood: A longitudinal follow-up, *Developmental Psychopathology,* 18:233–251.

Doesburg, S. M., Chau, C. M., Cheung, T.P.L., Moiseev, A, et al (2013), Neonatal pain-related stress, functional cortical activity and visual-perceptual abilities in school-age children born at extremely low gestational age, *Pain,* 154(10):1946–1952.

Drew, S. (2007). 'Having cancer changed my life, and changed my life forever': Survival, illness legacy and service provision following cancer in childhood, *Chronic Illness,* 3:278–295.

Dromi, E. (1987). *Early Lexical Development,* Cambridge: Cambridge University Press.

Edleson, J. L. (1999). Children's witnessing of adult domestic violence, *Journal of Interpersonal Violence,* 14:839–870.

Eliot, M., Cornell, D. G. (2009). Bullying in middle school as a function of insecure attachment and aggressive attitudes, *School Psychology International,* 30:201.

Erdos, C., Genesee, F., Savage, R., Haigh, C. A. (2010), Individual differences in second language reading outcomes, *International Journal of Bilingualism,* 15(1):3–25.

Espelage, D. L., Bosworth, K., Simon, T. (2000). Examining the social environment of middle school students who bully, *Journal of Counseling and Development,* 78:326–333.

Evans, S., de Souza, L. (2008). Dealing with chronic pain: Giving voice to the experiences of mothers with chronic pain and their children, *Qualitative Health Research,* 18(4):489–500.

Evans, S., Shipton, E. A., Keenan, T. (2006). The relationship between maternal chronic pain and child adjustment: The role of parenting as a mediator, *Journal of Pain,* 7:236–243.

Felitti, V. J., Anda, R. F., Nordenberg, D., Williamson, D. F., Spitz, A. M., et al (1998). Relationship of childhood abuse and household dysfunction to many of the leading causes of death in adults: The Adverse Childhood Experiences (ACE) study, *American Journal of Preventive Medicine,* 14(4):245–258.

Ferguson, K. S., Dacey, C. M. (1997). Anxiety, depression and dissociation in women health care providers reporting a history of childhood psychological abuse, *Child Abuse and Neglect,* 21(10):241–252.

Figley, C. R. (Ed) (1995). *Compassion Fatigue: Secondary Traumatic Stress Disorders from Treating the Traumatized,* New York: Brunner/Mazel.

Fogassi, L., Ferrarri, P. E. (2007). Mirror neurons and the evolution of embodied language, *Current Direction in Psychological Science,* 16(3):136–141.

Fonagy, P., Target, M. (1997). Attachment and reflective function: Their role in self-organization, *Development and Psychopathology,* 9:679–700.

Ford, J. D., Courtois, C. A. (2013). *Treating Traumatic Stress Disorders in Children and Adolescents: Scientific Foundations and Therapeutic Models,* New York: Guilford Press.

Fox, L., Long, S., Anglois, A. (1988). Patterns of language comprehension deficit in abused and neglected children, *Journal of Speech and Hearing Disorders,* (53):239–244.

Freyd, J. J., Birrell, P. (2013). *Blind To Betrayal: Why We Fool Ourselves We Aren't Being Fooled,* Hoboken, NJ, John Wiley and Sons.

Fuemmeler, B. F., Elkin, D. T., Mullins, L. L. (2002). Survivors of childhood brain tumors: Behavioral, emotional, and social adjustment, *Clinical Psychology Review,* 22:547–585.

Fuller-Thomson, E., Mehta, R., Valeo, A. (2014). Establishing a link between attention deficit disorder/attention deficit hyperactivity disorder and childhood physical abuse, *Journal of Aggression, Maltreatment & Trauma,* 23(2):188–198.

Gaensbauer, T. J. (2002). Representations of trauma in infancy: Clinical and theoretical implications for the understanding of early memory, *Infant Mental Health Journal,* 23(3):259–277.

Gaensbauer, T. J. (2011). Embodied simulation, mirror neurons, and the reenactment of trauma in early childhood, *Neuropsychoanalysis: An Interdisciplinary Journal for Psychoanalysis and the Neurosciences,* 13(1):91–107.

Gil, K. M., Williams, D. A., Thompson, R. J., Kinney, T. R. (1991). Sickle cell disease in children and adolescents: The relation of child and parent pain coping strategies to adjustment, *Journal of Pediatric Psychology,* 16:643–663.

Giovanni, L. (2004). Trauma, dissociation, and disorganized attachment: Three strands of a single braid, *Psychotherapy, Theory, Research, Practice, Training,* 41:472–86.

Gleason, J. B., Ratner, N. B. (2009). *The Development of Language,* 7th ed, New York: Pearson Education, Inc.

Goldson, E. (1998). Children with disabilities and child maltreatment, *Child Abuse & Neglect*, 22:663–667.

Gomez, A. (2012). *EMDR Therapy and Adjunct Approaches with Children: Complex Trauma, Attachment, and Dissociation*, New York: Springer Publishing Company.

Gray, D. G. (2002). *Attaching In Adoption: Practical Tools for Today's Parents*, Indianapolis: Perspectives Press.

Haapasalo, J., Aaltonen, P. (1999). Mothers' abusive childhood predicts child abuse, *Child Abuse Review*, 8(4):231–250.

Halla, S. (Ed) (1999). *The Development of Social Cognition*, Studies in Developmental Psychology Series. New York: Psychology Press.

Harding, E., Riley, P. (1986). *The Bilingual Family: A Handbook for Parents*, Cambridge: Cambridge University Press.

Hastings, R. P., Kovshoff, H., Brown, T., Ward, N. J., Degli Espinosa, F., Remington, B. (2005). Coping strategies in mothers and fathers of preschool and school-age children with autism, *Autism*, 9:377.

Heineman, T. V. (1998). *The Abused Child: Psychodynamic Understanding and Treatment*, New York: Guilford Press.

Heller, L., Lapierre, A. (2012). *Healing Developmental Trauma: How Early Trauma Affects Self-Regulation, Self-Image, and the Capacity for Relationship*, Berkeley, CA: North Atlantic Books.

Henninghausen, K., Lyons-Ruth, K. (2007). *Disorganization of Attachment Strategies in Infancy and Childhood; Encyclopedia on Early Childhood Development*, Montreal: Centre of Excellence for Early Childhood Development.

Herman, J. (1997). *Trauma and Recovery: The Aftermath of Violence—From Domestic Abuse to Political Terror*, New York: Basic Books.

Hershkowitz, I., Lamb, M. E., Horowitz, D. (2007). Victimization of children with disabilities, *American Journal Of Orthopsychiatry*, 77(4):629–635.

Heymann, K. L. (2010). *The Sound of Hope: Recognizing, Coping with, and Treating Your Child's Auditory Processing Disorder*, New York: Ballantine Books.

Hildyard, K. L., Wolfe, A. W. (2002). Child neglect: Developmental issues and outcomes, *Child Abuse & Neglect*, 26:679–695.

Hinduja, S., Patchin, J. W. (2010). Bullying, cyberbullying, and suicide, *Archives of Suicide Research*, 14(3):206–221.

Holt, S., Buckley, H., Whelan, S. (2008). The impact of exposure to domestic violence on children and young people: A review of the literature. *Child Abuse & Neglect*, 32:797–810.

Hough, S. D., Kaczmarek, L. (2011). Language and reading outcomes in young children adopted from Eastern European orphanages, *Journal of Early Intervention*, 33(1):51–74.

Howell, E. F. (2011). *Understanding and Treating Dissociative Identity Disorder: A Relational Approach*, Relational Perspectives Book Series, New York: Routledge.

ISSTD Child & Adolescent Committee (2004). Guidelines for the evaluation and treatment of dissociative symptoms in children and adolescents, *Journal of Trauma and Dissociation*, 5(3).

ISSTD Child & Adolescent Committee (2008). Frequently Asked Questions for Parents. International Society for the Study of Trauma and Dissociation, http://www.isst-d.org/education/faq-child.htm.

ISSTD Child & Adolescent Committee (2009). Frequently Asked Questions for Teachers. International Society for the Study of Trauma and Dissociation, http://www.isst-d.org/education/faq-teachers.htm.

ISSTD (2011). Guidelines for treating dissociative identity disorder in adults, Third Revision, *Journal of Trauma and Dissociation*, 12(2):115–187.

Jamora, M. S., Brylske, P. D., Martens, P., Braxton, D., Colantuoni, E., Belcher, H.M.E. (2009). Children in foster care: Adverse Childhood Experiences and psychiatric diagnoses, *Journal of Child & Adolescent Trauma*, 2(3):198–208.

Janus, M., Goldberg, S. (1997). Treatment characteristics of congenital heart disease and behavior problems of patients and healthy siblings, *Journal of Paediatrics and Child Health*, 33:219–225.

Johnson, B., Francis, J. (2005). Emotional and behavioural problems in children and adolescents with congenital heart disease, *Journal of Indian Association for Child and Adolescent Mental Health*, 1(4):Article 5.

Kagan, R. (2004). *Rebuilding Attachments with Traumatized Children: Healing from Losses, Violence, Abuse, and Neglect*, New York: Hayworth Press.

Kaminski, M., Pellino, T., Wish, J. (2002). Play and pets: The physical and emotional impact of child-life and pet therapy on hospitalized children, *Children's Health Care*, 31(4):321–335.

Kassam-Adams, N., Garcia-España, J. F., Fein, J. A., Winston, F. K. (2005). Heart rate and post-traumatic stress in injured children, *Archives of General Psychiatry*, 63:335–340.

Kazak, A. E., Kassam-Adams, N., Schneider, S., Zelikovsky, N. Alderfer, M. A., Rourke, M. (2006). An integrative model of pediatric medical traumatic stress, *Journal of Pediatric Psychology*, 31(4):343–355.

Kearney, C. A. (2006). *Casebook in Child Behavior Disorders*, 3rd ed, Belmont, CA: Thomson and Wadsworth.

Kendall-Tackett, K. (2002). The health effects of childhood abuse: Four pathways by which abuse can influence health, *Child Abuse & Neglect*, 6(7):715–730.

Kia-Keating, M., Ellis, B. H. (2007). Belonging and connection to school in resettlement: Young refugees, school belonging, and psychosocial adjustment, *Clinical Child Psychology and Psychiatry*, 12:29.

Kluft, R. P. (1985). Childhood multiple personality disorder: Predictors, clinical findings and treatment results. In R. P. Kluft (Ed.), *Childhood Antecedents of Multiple Personality Disorder*, Washington, DC: American Psychiatric Press.

Knickmeyer, R. C., Gouttard, S., Kang, C., Evans, D., Wilber, K., et al (2008). A structural MRI study of human brain development from birth to 2 years, *Journal of Neuroscience*, 28(47):12176–12182.

Knutson, J., Sullivan, P. (1993). Communicative disorders as a risk factor in abuse, *Topics in Language Disorders*, 13(4):1–14.

Konner, M. (2010). *The Evolution of Childhood: Relationships, Emotion, Mind*, Cambridge, MA: The Belknap Press of Harvard University Press.

Koomen, H. M., Hoeksma, J. B. (1993). Early hospitalization and disturbances of infant behaviour and the mother-infant relationship, *Journal of Child Psychology and Psychiatry*, 34:917–934.

Kurtz, P. D., Gaudin, J. M., Wodarski, J. S., Howing, P. T. (1993). Maltreatment and the school aged child: School performance consequences, *Child Abuse & Neglect*, 17:581–589.

Kuttner, L. (2010). *A Child in Pain: What Health Professionals Can Do to Help*, Carmarthen, Wales: Crown House Publishing.

Landry, S. H., Smith, K. E., Swank, P. R. (2006a). Responsive parenting: Establishing early foundations for social, communication, and independent problem-solving skills, *Developmental Psychology*, 42(4):627–642.

Landry, S. H., Swank, P. R., Smith, K. E., Assel, M. A., Gunnewig, S. B. (2006b). Enhancing early literacy skills for preschool children: Bringing a professional development model to scale, *Journal of Learning Disabilities*, 39:306–324.

Landy, S., Menna, R. (2001). Play between aggressive young children and their mothers, *Clinical Child Psychology and Psychiatry,* 6:223.

Lehman, C. (2005). *Strong at the Heart: How It Feels to Heal from Sexual Abuse,* New York: Melanie Kroupe Books, Farrar, Straus, and Giroux.

Leung, E., Tasker, S. L., Atkinson, L., Vaillancourt, T., Schulkin, J., Schmidt, L. A. (2010). Perceived maternal stress during pregnancy and its relation to infant stress reactivity at 2 days and 10 months of postnatal life, *Clinical Pediatrics,* 49(2):158–165.

Levendosky, A. A., Huth-Bocks, A. C., Shapiro, D. L., Semel, M. A. (2003). The impact of domestic violence on the maternal–child relationship and preschool-age children's functioning, *Journal of Family Psychology,* 17(3):275–287.

Levine, P. A., Kline, M. (2007). *Trauma through a Child's Eyes: Awakening the Ordinary Miracle of Healing,* Berkeley, CA: North Atlantic Books.

Levine, P. A., Maté, G. (2010). *In an Unspoken Voice: How the Body Releases Trauma and Restores Goodness,* Berkeley, CA: North Atlantic Books.

Liossi, C. (1999). Management of paediatric procedure-related cancer pain, *Pain Reviews,* 6:279–302.

Liotti, G. (2004). A model of dissociation based on attachment theory and research, *Psychotherapy: Theory, Research, Practice, Training,* 41:472–486.

Liotti, G. (2009). Attachment and dissociation. In P. F. Dell & J. O'Neill (Eds), *Dissociation: DSM-V and Beyond* (pp. 53–65), New York: Routledge Press.

Loewenstein, R. J. (2006). A hands-on clinical guide to the stabilization phase of dissociative identity disorder treatment, *Psychiatric Clinics of North America,* 29(1):305–333.

Lyons-Ruth, K., Block, D., (1996). The disturbed caregiving system: Relations among childhood trauma, maternal caregiving, and infant affect and attachment, *Infant Mental Health Journal,* 17(3):257–275.

Lyons-Ruth, K., Bureau, J. F., Riley, C. D., Atlas-Corbett, A. F. (2009). Socially indiscriminate attachment behavior in the Strange Situation: Convergent and discriminant validity in relation to caregiving risk, later behavior problems, and attachment insecurity, *Development and Psychopathology,* 21(2):355–372.

Lyons-Ruth, K., Durta, L., Shuder, M. R., Bianchi, I. (2006). From infant attachment disorganization to adult dissociation: Relational adaptations or traumatic experiences? *Psychiatric Clinics of North America,* 29(1):63–86.

Maciver, D., Jones, D., Nicol, M. (2010). Parents' experiences of caring for a child with chronic pain, *Qualitative Health Research,* 20(9):1272–1282.

Martin, R., Dombrowski, S. C. (2008). *Prenatal Exposures: Psychological and Educational Consequences for Children,* New York: Springer Science & Business Media.

Mashburn, A. J. (2008). Quality of social and physical environments in preschools and children's development of academic, language, and literacy skills, *Applied Developmental Science,* 12(3):113–127.

Mashburn, A. J., Pianta, R. C., Hamre, B. K., Downer, J. T., Barbarin, et al (2008). Measures of classroom quality in prekindergarten and children's development of academic, language, and social skills, *Child Development,* 79(3):732–749.

Mathieu, F. (2011). *The Compassion Fatigue Workbook: Creative Tools for Transforming Compassion Fatigue and Vicarious Traumatization,* Psychosocial Stress Series, New York: Routledge.

May, L., Byers-Heinlein, K., Gervain, J., Werker, J. F. (2011). Language and the newborn brain: Does prenatal language experience shape the neonate neural response to speech? *Frontiers in Psychology: Language Sciences,* 2:Article 222.

McAleer Hamaguchi, P. (2001). *Childhood Speech, Language & Listening Problems: What Every Parent Should Know,* 2nd Edition, New York: John Wiley & Sons (Part 3).

Merriam Webster Dictionary, an Encyclopedia Britannica Company: http://www.merriam-webster.com/

Mikkelsson, M., Sourander, A., Piha, J., Salminen, J. J. (1997). Psychiatric symptoms in pre-adolescents with musculoskeletal pain and fibromyalgia, *Pediatrics,* 100(2):220–227.

Miller, L. C. (2005). *The Handbook of International Adoption Medicine: A Guide for Physicians, Parents, and Providers,* New York: Oxford University Press.

Milot, T., St-Laurent, D., Éthier, L. S., Provost, M. A. (2010). Trauma-related symptoms in neglected preschoolers and affective quality of mother-child communication, *Child Maltreatment,* 15:293.

Nabors, L. A., Weist, M. D., Shugarman, R., Woeste, M. J., Mullet, E., Rosner, L. (2004). Assessment, prevention, and intervention activities in a school-based program for children experiencing homelessness, *Behavior Modification,* 28:565.

Nadeau, M. E., Nolin, P. (2013). Attentional and executive functions in neglected children, *Journal of Child & Adolescent Trauma,* 6(1).

Nadeau , M. E., Nolin, P., Chartrand, C. (2013). Behavioral and emotional profiles of neglected children, *Journal of Child & Adolescent Trauma,* 6(1):11–24.

Nader, K., Salloum, A. (2011). Complicated grief reactions in children and adolescents, *Journal of Child & Adolescent Trauma,* 4(3):233–257.

Nazzi, T., Bertoncini, J., Mehler, J. (1998). Language discrimination by newborns: Toward an understanding of the role of rhythm, *Journal of Experimental Psychology: Human Perception and Performance,* 24:756–766.

Nelson, C. A. (1987). The recognition of facial expressions in the first two years of life: Mechanisms of development, *Child Development,* 58(4):889–909.

Netherton, S. D., Holmes, D., Walker, C. E. (1999). *Child and Adolescent Psychological Disorders,* Oxford: Oxford University Press.

Newacheck, P. W., Taylor, W. R. (1992). Childhood chronic illness: Prevalence, severity, and impact, *American Journal of Public Health,* 82:364–371.

Newberry, R. C., Swanson, J. C. (2008). Implications of breaking mother–young social bonds, *Applied Animal Behavior Science,* 10(1–2):3–23.

Nijenhuis, E.R.S. (2004). *Somatoform Dissociation: Phenomena, Measurement, and Theoretical Issues,* New York: Norton.

Ninio, A., Snow, C. (1996). *Pragmatic Development,* Boulder, CO: Westview Press.

Nippold, M. A. (2007). *Later Language Development: School-Aged Children, Adolescents, and Young Adults,* 3rd ed, Austin, TX: Pro-Ed.

Ødegård, W. (2005). Chronic illness as a challenge to the attachment process, *Clinical Child Psychology and Psychiatry,* 10:13.

Orbach, I. (1988). *Children Who Don't Want to Live: Understanding and Treating the Suidical Child,* San Francisco: Jossey-Bass.

O'Shea, B., Hodes, M., Down, G., Bramley, J. (2000). A school-based mental health service for refugee children, *Clinical Child Psychology and Psychiatry,* 5:189.

Osofsky, J. D. (Ed) (2011). *Clinical Work with Traumatized Young Children,* New York: Guilford Press.

Ostrowski, S. A., Norman, M. A., Christopher, C., Delahanty, D. L. (2007). Brief report: The impact of maternal posttraumatic stress disorder symptoms and child gender on risk for persistent posttraumatic stress disorder symptoms in child trauma victims, *Journal of Pediatric Psychology,* 32(3):338–342.

Pearce, J. W., Pezzot-Pearce, T. D. (1997). *Psychotherapy of Abused and Neglected Children*, New York: Guilford Press.

Pearlman, L. A., Saakvitne, K. W. (1995). *Trauma and the Therapist: Countertransference and Vicarious Traumatization in Psychotherapy with Incest Survivors*, New York: W. W. Norton.

Perez, C. M., Widom, C. S. (1994). Childhood victimization and long-term intellectual and academic outcomes, *Child Abuse & Neglect*, 18:617–633.

Perry, B. D., Szalavitz, M. (2006). *The Boy Who Was Raised as A Dog and Other Stories from a Child Psychiatrist's Notebook: What Traumatized Children Can Teach Us about Loss, Love, and Healing*, New York: Basic Books.

Piazza, C. C., Carroll-Hernandez, T. A. (2004). Assessment and treatment of pediatric feeding disorders, *Encyclopedia on Early Childhood Development*, Montreal: Centre of Excellence for Early Childhood Development.

Pillai Riddell, R. R., Stevens, B. J., McKeever, P., Gibbins, S., Asztalos, L., Katz, J. (2009). Chronic pain in hospitalized infants: Health professionals' perspectives, *Journal of Pain*, 10(12):1217–1225.

Pollak, S. D., Cicchetti, D., Hornung, K., Reed, A. (2000). Recognizing emotion in faces: Developmental effects of child abuse and neglect, *Developmental Psychology*, 36:679–688.

Putnam, F. W. (1993). Dissociation in the inner city. In R. P. Kluft & C. G. Fine (Eds), *Clinical Perspectives on Multiple Personality Disorder* (pp. 179–200). Washington, DC: American Psychiatric Publishing.

Putnam, F. W. (1997). *Dissociation in Children and Adolescents: A Developmental Perspective*. New York: Guilford Press.

Quin Yow, W., Markman, E. M. (2011). Young bilingual children's heightened sensitivity to referential cues, *Journal of Cognition and Development*, 12(1):12–31.

Redmond, S. M. (2002). The use of rating scales with children who have language impairments, *American Journal of Speech Language Pathology*, 11:124–138.

Rizzolatti, G., Craighero, L. (2004). The mirror-neuron system, *Annual Review of Neuroscience*, 27:169–192.

Robson, L. M., Leung, A.K.C., Thomason, M. A. (2006). Catheterization of the bladder in infants and children, *Clinical Pediatrics*, 45:795.

Rogers, S. J., Williams, J.H.G. (Eds) (2006). *Imitation and the Social Mind: Autism and Typical Development*, New York: Guilford Press.

Rothchild, B. (2006). *Help for the Helper: The Psychophysiology of Compassion Fatigue and Vicarious Trauma*, New York: Norton Professional Books.

Saakvitne, K. W., Pearlman, L. A. (1996). *Transforming the Pain: A Workbook on Vicarious Trauma*, New York: Norton Professional Books.

Saxe, G. N., Stoddard, F., Hall, E., Chawla, N., Lopez, C., Sheridan, R. (2005). Pathways to PTSD, part I: Children with burns. *American Journal of Psychiatry*, 162:1299–1304.

Scaer, R. (2014). *The Body Bears the Burden: Trauma, Dissociation, and Disease*, 3rd ed, New York: Routledge.

Schaefer, C. E., Gitlin, K., Sandgrund, A. (1991). *Play Diagnosis and Assessment*. New York: Wiley.

Schäfer, I., Barkmann, C., Riedesser, P., Schulte-Markwort, M. (2004). Peritraumatic dissociation predicts posttraumatic stress in children and adolescents following road traffic accidents, *Journal of Trauma & Dissociation*, 5(4):79–92.

Scherr, T. G. (2007). Educational experiences of children in foster care: Meta-analyses of special education, retention and discipline rates, *School Psychology International*, 28:419.

Schiefelbusch, R. L. (Ed.) (1986). *Language Competence: Assessment and Intervention*. San Diego: College-Hill Press.

Schore, A. N. (2001). The early effects of trauma on right brain development, affect regulation and infant health, *Infant Mental Health Journal*, 22:201–269.

Schore, A. N. (2012). *The Science of the Art of Psychotherapy*, Norton Series on Interpersonal Neurobiology, New York: W. W. Norton & Company.

Schwartz, A. (2013). A.D.H.D. experts re-evaluate study's zeal for drugs, *New York Times*, New York edition, December 30, 2013, page A11.

Schwartz, A. (2014). Thousands of toddlers are medicated for A.D.H.D., report finds, raising worries, *New York Times*, New York edition, May 17, 2014, page A11.

Schwartz, H. L. (2000). *Dialogues with Forgotten Voices: Relational Perspectives on Child Abuse, Trauma, and Treatment of Dissociative Disorders,* New York: Basic Books.

Shaw, R. J., Deblois, T., Ikuta, L., Ginzburg, K., Fleisher, B., Koopman, C. (2006). Acute stress disorder among parents of infants in the neonatal intensive care nursery, *Psychosomatics*, 47:206–212.

Shields, A., Cicchetti, D. (1998). Reactive aggression among maltreated children: The contributions of attention and emotion dysregulation, *Journal of Clinical Child Psychology*, 27:381–395.

Shiminski-Maher, T. (1993). Physician-patient-parent communication problems, *Pediatric Neurosurgery*, 19(2):104–108.

Shirar, L. (1996). *Dissociative Children: Bridging the Inner and Outer Worlds.* New York: Norton.

Siegel, D. A. (2012). *The Developing Mind: How Relationships and the Brain Interact to Shape Who We Are,* 2nd ed., New York: Guilford Press.

Silberg, J. L. (1998). *The Dissociative Child: Diagnoses, Treatment, and Management,* 2nd ed., Lutherville, MD: Sidran Press.

Silberg, J. L. (2013). *The Child Survivor: Helping Developmental Trauma and Dissociation,* New York: Routledge.

Siller, M., Sigman, M. (2002). The behaviors of parents of children with autism predict the subsequent development of their children's communication, *Journal of Autism and Developmental Disorders*, 32(2):77–89.

Siller, M., Sigman, M. (2008). Modeling longitudinal change in the language abilities of children with autism: Parent behaviors and child characteristics as predictors of change, *Developmental Psychology*, 44:1691–1704.

Silva, R. R. (Ed.) (2004). *Posttraumatic Stress Disorders in Children and Adolescents,* New York: Norton.

Simons, S.H.P., van Dijk, M., Anand, K. S., Roofthooft, D., van Lingen, R. A., Tibboel, D. (2003). Do we still hurt newborn babies? A prospective study of procedural pain and analgesia in neonates, *Archives of Pediatric and Adolescent Medicine,* 157:1058–1064.

Smith, K. A., Gouze, K. R. (2004). *The Sensory-Sensitive Child: Practical Solutions for Out-of-Bounds Behavior*, New York: Harper Resource, Harper Collins.

Smith, S. L., Howard, J. A., Monroe, A. D. (1998). An analysis of child behavior problems in adoptions in difficulty, *Journal of Social Service Research*, 24(1–2):6–84.

Sousa, C., Herrenkohl, T. I., Moylan, C. A., Tajima A. E., Klika, J. B., et al (2011). Longitudinal study on the effects of child abuse and children's exposure to domestic violence, parent–child attachments, and antisocial behavior in adolescence, *Journal of Interpersonal Violence*, 26(1):111–136.

Speechley, K. N., Noh, S. (1992). Surviving childhood cancer, social support, and parents' psychological adjustment, *Journal of Pediatric Psychiatry*, 17:15–31.

Sprang, G., Katz, D. A., Cooke, C. (2009). Allostatic load: Considering the burden of cumulative trauma on children in foster care, *Journal of Child & Adolescent Trauma*, 2(4):242–252.

Stafstrom, C. E., Rostasy, K., Minster, A. (2002). The usefulness of children's drawings in the diagnosis of headache, *Pediatrics,* 109:460–472.

Stams, G.J.J.M., Juffer, F., van Ijzendoorn, M. H. (2002). Maternal sensitivity, infant attachment, and temperament in early childhood predict adjustment in middle childhood: The case of adopted children and their biologically unrelated parents, *Developmental Psychology,* 38:806–821.

Steinberg, M., Schnall, M. (2000). *The Stranger in the Mirror: Dissociation—The Hidden Epidemic,* New York: Harper-Collins.

Stien, P. T., Kendall, J. (2004). *Psychological Trauma and the Developing Brain: Neurologically Based Interventions for Troubled Children.* New York: Hayworth Press.

Stolbach, B. C., Minshew, R., Rompala, V., Dominguez R. Z., Gazibara, T., Fink, R. (2013). Complex trauma exposure and symptoms in urban traumatized children: A preliminary test of proposed criteria for developmental trauma disorder, *Journal of Traumatic Stress,* 25–26(4):483–491.

Strong, M. (1999). *A Bright Red Scream: Self-Mutilation and the Language of Pain,* New York, Penguin Books.

Suits, K., Tulviste, T., Ong, R., Tulviste, J., Kolk, A. (2011). Differences between humor comprehension and appreciation in healthy children and children with epilepsy, *Journal of Child Neurology,* 1:9.

Sullivan, P. M., Brookhouser, P. E., Scanlan, J. M., Knutson, J. F., Schulte, L. E. (1991). Patterns of physical and sexual abuse of communicatively handicapped children, *Annals of Otology, Rhinology & Laryngology,* 100:188–194.

Sullivan, P. M., Knutson, J. F. (1998). The association between child maltreatment and disabilities in a hospital-based epidemiological study, *Child Abuse & Neglect,* 22:271–288.

Sullivan, P. M., Knutson, J. F. (2000). Maltreatment and disabilities: A population-based epidemiological study, *Child Abuse & Neglect,* 24:1257–1274.

Sullivan, P. M., Knutson, J. F., Ashford, E. J. (2009). Maltreatment of children and youth with special healthcare needs. In A. P. Giardino, M. A. Lyn, E. R. Giardino (Eds) *A Practical Guide to the Evaluation of Child Physical Abuse and Neglect* (pp. 335–351), New York: Springer.

Sullivan, P. M., Vernon, M., Scanlan, J. M. (1987). Sexual abuse of deaf youth, *American Annals of the Deaf,* 32(4):256–262.

Sussman, F. (1999). *More Than Words: Helping Parents Promote Communication and Social Skills in Children with Autism Spectrum Disorder.* Toronto: The Hanen Centre.

Takizawa, R., Maughan, B., Arseneault, L. (2014). Adult health outcomes of childhood bullying victimization, evidence from a five-decade longitudinal British birth cohort, *American Journal of Psychiatry,* 171(7):777–784.

Talamas, A., Kroll, J. F., Dufour, R. (1999). From form to meaning: Stages in the acquisition of second-language vocabulary. *Bilingualism: Language and Cognition,* 2(1):45–58.

Teicher, M. H., Dumont, N. L., Ito, Y., Vaituzis, C., Giedd, J. N., Andersen, S. L. (2004). Childhood neglect is associated with reduced corpus callosum area, *Biological Psychiatry,* 56(2):80–85.

Terr, L.(1983). Time sense following psychic trauma: A clinical study of ten adults and twenty children, *American Journal of Orthopsychiatry,* 53:211–261.

Terr, L. (1990). *Too Scared to Cry: Psychic Trauma in Childhood,* New York: Basic Books.

Thompson, B. L., Levitt, P., Stanwood, G. D. (2009). Prenatal exposure to drugs: Effects on brain development and implications for policy and education, *Science and Society: Nature Reviews: Neuroscience,* 10:303–312.

Tufnell, G. (2003). Refugee children, trauma and the law, *Clinical Child Psychology and Psychiatry,* 8:431.

US-DHHS. (2013a). *Child Maltreatment 2012,* Washington, DC: Administration for Children and Families, Administration on Children, Youth and Families, Children's Bureau.

US Department of Health and Human Services, Health Resources and Services Administration, Maternal and Child Health Bureau (2013b). *Child Health USA 2013.* Rockville, MD: US Department of Health and Human Services.

Vanderbilt, D., Young, R., MacDonald, H. Z., Grant-Knight, W., Saxe, G., Zuckerman, B. (2008). Asthma severity and PTSD symptoms among inner-city children: A pilot study, *Journal of Trauma & Dissociation,* 9(2):191–207.

van der Hart, O., Nijenhuis, E.R.S., Steele, K. (2006). *The Haunted Self: Structural Dissociation and the Treatment of Chronic Traumatization.* New York: Norton.

van der Kolk, B. A. (2005). Developmental trauma disorder: Towards a rational diagnosis for children with complex trauma histories, *The Psychiatric Annals,* 35(5):401–408.

van der Kolk, B. A. (2014). *The Body Keeps the Score: Brain, Mind and Body in the Healing of Trauma.* New York: Viking.

Varni, J. W., Rapoff, M. A., Waldron, S. A., Gragg, R. A., Bernstein, B. H., Lindsley, C. B. (1996). Chronic pain and emotional distress in children and adolescents, *Developmental and Behavioral Pediatrics,* 17(3):154–161.

Vissing, Y. M., Straus, M. A., Gelles, R. J., Harrop, J. W. (1991). Verbal aggression by parents and psychosocial problems of children, *Child Abuse and Neglect,* 15:223–238.

Vouloumanos, A., Werker, J. F. (2007). Listening to language at birth: Evidence for a bias for speech in neonates, *Developmental Science,* 10:159–164.

Wallin, D. J. (2007). *Attachment in Psychotherapy,* New York: Guilford Press.

Waters, F. (2005). When treatment fails with traumatized children . . . Why? *Journal of Trauma and Dissociation,* 6:1–9.

Wieland, S. (Ed) (2011). *Dissociation in Traumatized Children and Adolescents: Theory and Clinical Interventions,* Psychological Stress Series, New York: Routledge.

William T., Zempsky, W. T., Cravero, J. P., Committee on Pediatric Emergency Medicine and Section on Anesthesiology and Pain Medicine (2004). Relief of pain and anxiety in pediatric patients in emergency medical systems. Clinical report: Guidance for the clinician in rendering pediatric care, *Pediatrics,* 114:1348–1356.

Winston, F. K., Kassam-Adams, N., Vivarelli-O'Neill, C., Ford, J., Newman, E., et al. (2002). Acute stress disorder symptoms in children and their parents after pediatric traffic injury, *Pediatrics,* 109:e90.

Wintgens, A., Boileau, B., Robaey, P. (1997). Posttraumatic stress symptoms and medical procedures in children, *Canadian Journal of Psychiatry,* 42:611–616.

Wodarski, J. S., Kurtz, P. D., Gaudin, J. M. Jr., Howling, P. T. (1990). Maltreatment and the school-aged child: Major academic, socioemotional, and adaptive outcomes. *Social Work,* 35(6):506–513.

World Health Organization (2013). *Guidelines on the Pharmacological Treatment of Persisting Pain in Children with Medical Illnesses,* Persisting Pain in Children package, Geneva: WHO Library.

Yehuda, N. (2004). Critical issues: Dissociation in schoolchildren: An epidemic of failing in disguise. *International Society for the Study of Dissociation News,* 22:8–9.

Yehuda, N. (2005). The language of dissociation. *Journal of Trauma and Dissociation,* 6:9–29.

Yehuda, N. (2011). Leroy (7 years old)—"It is almost like he is two children": Working with a dissociative child in a school setting. In S. Wieland (Ed) *Dissociation in Traumatized Children and Adolescents: Theory and Clinical Interventions,* Psychological Trauma Series, New York: Routledge.

Yehuda, R., Mulherin Engel, S., Brand, S. R., Seckl, J., Marcus, S. M., Berkowitz, G. S. (2005). Transgenerational effects of posttraumatic stress disorder in babies of mothers exposed to the World Trade Center attacks during pregnancy, *Journal of Clinical Endocrinology & Metabolism,* 90(7):4115–4118.

Yehuda, R., Teicher, M. H., Seckl, J. R., Grossman, R. A., Morris, A., Bierer, L. M. (2007). Parental posttraumatic stress disorder as a vulnerability factor for low cortisol trait in offspring of Holocaust survivors, *Archives of General Psychiatry,* 64(9):1040–1048.

Yoder, P. J., Warren, S. F. (2002). Effects of prelinguistic milieu teaching and parent responsivity education on dyads involving children with intellectual disabilities, *Journal of Speech, Language, and Hearing Research,* 45:1158–1174.

Ziegler, M. F. Greenwald, M. H., DeGuzman, M. A., Simon, H. K. (2005). Posttraumatic stress responses in children: Awareness and practice among a sample of pediatric emergency care providers, *Pediatrics,* 115:1261–1267.

Zimrin, H. (1986). A profile of survival, *Child Abuse & Neglect,* 10(3):339–349.

Index